AF691749

And so on.

This is what most dentists will do—make assumptions. Is that who you are? The *average* "herd animal?" Are you a "change coward?" (If you fail to creatively confront change, change *will* confront you!)

The wise dentist will investigate. Get all the facts. Get the (complimentary) analysis and Financial Forecast for his practice. Ask questions. Come to an independent decision. Is that who you are?

If so, you can take a completely safe and informative next step by scheduling a private Discovery Call.

(If you are already a "major league player," doing very well but eager to do even better, you can jump the line and place a call to me, Parthiv Shah, directly at 301-873-5791. Or go to: ***MeetParthiv.com*** *and book your appointment. I am a CEO, but then, so are you! So, I am accessible.)*

MY MISSION IS SIMPLE AND STRAIGHTFORWARD.

1: To help dentists have much better practices and lives.
2: To be clearly, measurably worth a lot more than I "cost" or be fired.
3: To find dentists I am certain we can work for and with SUCCESSFULLY, and screen out others. We have no purpose but to be helpful and valuable. **YOU NEED NOT FEAR US!** Because we live on a month-to-month basis, there is NO benefit to us to just "make a sale". We MUST say "No" to some dentists. We MUST use our analytics to *identify who we will succeed with in advance.*

The trouble with a regular practice is, to use a business term, unit of sale or transaction size.

TO REACH EACH MILLION DOLLARS IN NET NEW REVENUE

FULL-MOUTH MAKEOVER @ $25,000	42 patients
SINGLE ARCH @ $12,000	84 patients
SINGLE TOOTH IMPLANT @ $6,000	167 patients
SINGLE REG. DDS. APPOINTMENT @ $165	6,000 patients!

The smaller the unit of sale, the more units are needed for each income goal—and with that more patients and new patients, more advertising, more staff, more hours of work...more anxiety and stress and weariness.

This can't really be fixed in an ordinary practice. It can be fixed by "re-engineering" the practice to be much more about implant dentistry.

This can be done for you!

If it happens to be true that you are behind in accumulating wealth for exit/retirement and security, you can make up ground much faster with $25,0000 and $50,000 units of sale than with $3,000 or $1,000.

And what of the value of your practice? Will you let the equity and value of your practice, a life's work, be ruined? The consolidators' plan is to diminish the value of general dental practices so as to buy them as bargains or simply force their closure*. But, if you re-engineer your practice to be markedly unordinary...with "more from fewer and less" and with a functioning System of generating high unit-of-sale patients/cases, a System exclusive to you...you can thwart their diabolical plan!

*One of the biggest corporate consolidators recently endowed a new dental college at a university with $100 million of support, putting them in front of everybody else in having those students as interns, then hiring them, so as to "turn over" the dentists in the practices they own, buy and operate and staff with young, lower cost dentists. They have a "vision" for general dentistry and it does not include top compensation for dentists! YOUR future is in YOUR hands! Protecting it requires action, now.

Read This ONLY IF You Consider Yourself A "BIG Thinker"

There is an option to make an even bigger, grander leap to a "new breed" of dental practice with our Comprehensive Dental Practice Growth Machine. It includes Sell-More-Implants™ plus much more, depending on your situation, interests and clinical capabilities. There is a Sell-More-SYSTEM for sedation dentistry, perio-gum disease treatment, cosmetic, sleep, etc.

You can decide whether to ask about it during your Discovery Call. Here are a few thoughts to help that consideration:

Question: Isn't it about time you decide you deserve top-level financial success and security?
This is being taken away from you, bit by bit by bit.

By insurers. "Brand," corporate dental retail chains moving in and dominating with advertising. Rising staffing costs and other inflation. Maybe also recent investment losses or at least inability for saved money to grow.

The results of this are terrible. You having to work harder, struggle to bring in more new patients, suppress fees, accept less net take-home income, *and push the retirement goal posts further away.* This has you frustrated and disappointed, and your spouse and family frustrated and disappointed. Plans made are stalled. Promises made to yourself and to your spouse can't be kept. This is not what you signed up for, is it?

There is only one practical solution. Cost-cutting within the practice has its limits—and you may already have reached them. Taking home less money and investing less money is an answer, but obviously not a solution. **This set of circumstances has but one cure: a lot more income—without proportionately increasing overhead and without working yourself to death.**

INCREMENTALISM OR TRANSFORMATION?

Most dentists do not have the courage to really change. They act incrementally, trying to improve (or repair) one thing this month, another a few months later, circling and poking at their situation. How has that worked out? Breakthroughs do not happen incrementally. Ford didn't transform transportation with faster horses or diapers on horses. Come forward through all the history of business and industry and the same point is true. And at the small business level and with individuals and their lives, breakthroughs do *not* happen incrementally. *Something* ***big and bold has to be done to produce a big result.***

Somewhat remarkably, in this case you have the luxury of gradual transformation. We can add new/additional particular-need, high-value patients at a manageable pace you decide on. You can gradually increase your specialized work while decreasing your regular work, by cutting back on online or other advertising to attract ordinary new patients, by raising fees and intentionally sending lowest value patients elsewhere. This need *not* be a volcanic, disruptive, anxiety-producing transformation. Not at all! It can be measured and paced. But it can also lead to literally replacing your current practice with a new, different, better, more profitable, more financially efficient and more valuable practice.

You have a successful practice. But it's not unusual to have wound up creating and building a kind of success that is ultimately more of a trap and more of a source of stress and anxiety than you envisioned. The writer Oscar Wilde once said, ruefully, *"I'd quit writing but I can't, I'm too famous."* In this way, success can actually, ironically, become a form of failure! It's not too late. You can keep the best parts and aspects of your practice but replace the fragile, stressful, income limiting aspects. **THE DENTAL GROWTH MACHINE™** keeps and strengthens the practice but changes the patients and re-engineers the finances. Look into this!

Let's talk! Sincerely,

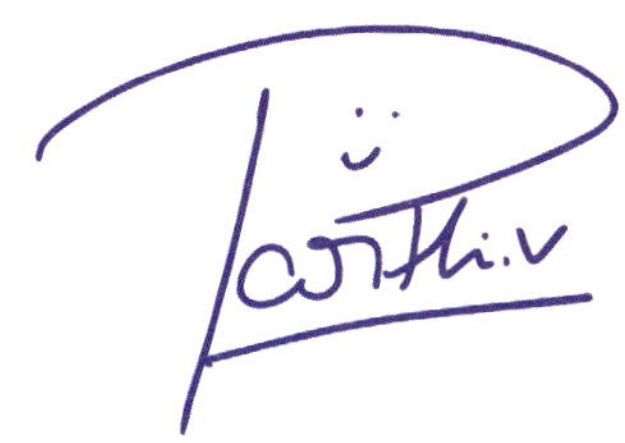

Parthiv Shah

Introduction

This book aims to help you take your practice to the next level...and then the next after that. If you're fresh out of dental school or just starting a new practice, man, I can't tell you how glad I am you're reading this right now. This book will allow you to bypass years of 60- to 70-hour weeks spent slaving away at the dentist's chair or, worse, being forced to send staff home early day after day because there are not enough patients coming in for treatment.

If you're already an established practice owner looking to achieve the level of success you dreamed of when you first chose this profession, then once again, I'm glad you're here. Selling more dental implants and high-end dental services will be a game changer. On average, a dentist needs SIX THOUSAND ordinary dental patients to equal the net revenue of 165 to 170 implant patients.

When you implement the proven strategies you're about to discover, you'll likely be booked weeks, if not months, in advance with high-end dental patients who eagerly seek you out and are excited to pay for and receive life-changing dental implants.

Whether you're just starting out or are a seasoned practice owner, I urge you to use this book as your business bible. Follow the steps outlined. Pay close attention to the examples. Learn how dentists who started off frustrated and barely getting by now operate multimillion-dollar practices. More importantly, learn how to completely revolutionize your practice in the next 12 to 18 months and go from an average dentist's office to a wealth-generating machine.

Why Choose Dentistry in the First Place?

Many of my clients tell me they chose to become dentists after experiencing the life-changing effects of dentistry in their own lives. As children or young adults, they were unhappy with their smiles. They had crooked teeth or had lost teeth due to trauma.

After renewing their smiles with the power of braces, dental implants, or the like, they felt that surge of confidence that comes with a radiant smile. Some watched loved ones with severe orthodontic concerns get out of pain and gain a new lease on life after restoring their teeth and smiles. They witnessed or experienced these transformations firsthand, and just knew...dentistry was for them.

They went to dental school because they wanted to relieve pain, improve esthetics and enhance the lives of the people who would grow to depend on them. They went to dental school because it seemed like a stable career, one with a respectable, if not sizable, income. Ultimately, they chose dentistry to make a difference in their patients' lives while supporting a comfortable, if not prosperous, lifestyle.

All the Right Reasons, But All the Wrong Results

Most new dentists start with stars in their eyes and the expectation of doing good for their patients and making a lot of money. Then reality hits.

Their years devoted to their profession and education landed them a 60- to70-hour per week job that, on average, pays about as well as an experienced plumber or mechanic.

These highly qualified individuals leave dental school often burdened with significant student loan debt exceeding $200,000. If they choose to go into business on their own, it's not uncommon to take out loans to cover the high overhead costs of owning a practice. As a practice owner, you must cover the costs of dental equipment, office space, staff salaries, utilities and liability insurance, to name a few. These costs eat into your revenue and make managing day-to-day operations and maintaining profitability a challenge.

Then, there are the typical problems most business owners face with competition and market saturation. It seems many towns have dental practices on every other corner—and most dentists have no idea how to set themselves apart from their competitors and attract enough high-end dental patients to be profitable.

The demanding nature of this profession, combined with the pressure of managing debt and overhead, takes a toll on your mental health. That stress and the long hours lead to burnout, anxiety and depression.

Not the future you had in mind when you chose dentistry, is it?

I bet not. Now, bear with me. The picture gets darker before we reveal the light, but I promise, there IS light at the end. That's why you're reading this, right? Because you know with the right strategies in place, you can take your career and your practice far above average and achieve the type of success you expected when you first chose dentistry. I promise all that is to come, but before diving into the good part, we must cover one more concern. Recently, we all lived through a nightmare scenario that challenged every business owner and dealt some industries a devastating blow. Some owners were driven out of business, while others are still working to recover. You probably already know where I'm going with this: back to 2020 and COVID-19.

Dentistry Disrupted: How COVID-19 Forever Changed Dentistry

Dental offices suffered a double punch from COVID. Most were forced to only provide emergency services and strictly limit their operations during lockdown. Others were forced to shut down entirely due to their own health concerns. When lockdowns eased, many dentists were forced to close their operations for good when, out of fear of infection, many of their patients did not return.

To this day, dentists report the fear-induced decrease has never completely righted itself. Market research backs this, showing that while dental patient influx has increased in the past years, it's still not back at pre-pandemic levels.

The next blow was felt by us all—skyrocketing inflation, which has increased the price of everything from cotton balls and scalpels to electricity and insurance. To make this worse, worldwide supply chain disruptions have led to delays and shortages of dental supplies and equipment. These supply chain disruptions cause scarcity in the market, which drives prices up even higher.

The economic fallout of the pandemic and current all-time high inflation rates have hit consumers as well, with many choosing to conserve their recourses and hold off on what they consider "elective procedures." This means raising prices is not an option for most dentists whose patients are unable or unwilling to afford even basic services.

This perfect storm of fewer patients wanting to pay for services, the rising costs of doing business, skyrocketing inflation, and new economic threats on the front page of every financial publication have driven many established dental practices out of business.

Ok. That's the end of the bad news, I promise!

Now, it's time to speak of solutions. Now, it's time to discuss how some dental practices, faced with the same industry challenges as the rest, are currently experiencing their most profitable years to date. Now, it's time to reveal how these thriving practice owners used strategic marketing to focus on attracting a hoard of high-value patients who are eager to say yes to dental implants and invest in high-end dental procedures. By doing this, they permanently removed their shackles from the dental chair. They created the dental practice of their dreams, one that runs like a well-oiled machine—one that runs whether the owner is there five days a week or vacationing at a secluded tropical paradise with unpredictable phone service and non-existent internet.

These savvy entrepreneurs are no longer forced to work long hours, nights and weekends to remain profitable. Many work far less than before and enjoy profits five or 10 times greater than in previous years. They achieved this success by following the advice you now have access to in this book. They achieved this level of success by adopting a business growth strategy and marketing system tailored to their practice. The dentists I work with have generated more than $50 million in dental implant and All-on-4 business over the past decade. These practice owners now operate at a new level. They have a business that works for them, with automation streamlining everything from marketing to customer retention and referrals to internal systems and procedures and more.

In this book, I provide specific details and insider strategies on how to take your practice from where it is now, even if it's barely out of the red, to higher gross revenue than you may have ever dreamed possible. I'll reveal how, with strategic guidance and automated marketing systems, you can grow your practice from a meager few hundred thousand in gross revenue to more than $2 million a year in the next 12 months. For the true entrepreneur, this is just the beginning. I've helped dozens of practice owners grow from $2 million to as high as $8 million or even $12 million in gross revenue over a 12-to-18-month period. The secrets of how I accomplished this are in this book.

How to Use This Book as Your Guide to Higher Profits with Dental Implants

In the chapters to come, I'll go into detail about the specific strategies I use to help practice owners become more profitable.

In the first chapter, I'll show you how to develop your comprehensive growth strategy. This is a personalized plan for measurable and consistent growth. We'll discuss how to use your well-crafted marketing message. Combining print and digital assets can supercharge your ability to educate and entice potential patients. An educated patient who understands why dental implants and high-end dental procedures are an investment in their health and confidence—one that protects their teeth, mouth and overall health—is more likely to agree to treatment.

> Your marketing message can be delivered digitally and at the click of a button when you have the right automation systems in place. With the right list of prospects, direct mail marketing can set you apart from other dental practices as the trusted go-to expert on dental implants, All-on-4s and high-end dental services.

I'll also discuss the Dental Data Protocol—the first step in transforming your practice. With Dental Data Protocol, I'll show you how to dive deep into your practice. We'll examine your current operating methods, practice procedures, marketing efforts and automation systems. We'll identify your processes for managing leads and current and past clients. Once we have a clear idea of how your practice is currently operating, we'll talk strategy.

I'll lay out the tactics you'll need to gather leads and successfully convert those leads into enthusiastic patients. We'll get into how to use automated systems to build and nurture lasting and profitable relationships with your patients and how to get those patients continuously referring their friends and family to you. By the end of this chapter, you should have a clear understanding of your current operations and an idea of what steps you should take next.

I'll discuss the most important elements of a successful marketing campaign: matching the right message to the right market. This chapter is all about having the right list of prospects, having something those prospects will benefit from, and then matching your prospect to what you offer with a marketing message that delivers an irresistible offer: A message designed to speak to patients who can afford dental implants, All-on-4s, and high-end dental services with or without the assistance of insurance.

This starts by identifying patients most likely to say yes. These patients may come from your current customer list or outside sources. Part of what makes me so good at what I do is identifying those most likely to benefit from what you offer and who can afford it. I am particularly skilled in identifying these markets for dentists and practice owners.

Once you've identified your ideal patient and developed your list of qualified leads, it's time to craft your message. For a marketing message to be effective, it has to offer compelling reasons your ideal patients should say yes to dental implants with your practice. This means they must understand how they will benefit from your services and why having their dental implant procedure done with you is in their best interest. Then, there needs to be an element of urgency; why do they need to start their dental implant or high-end dental procedures right away? Your message must convince your ideal prospects that it's in their best interest to say yes to the services or procedures you recommend as quickly as possible and that your practice is the only place they should have the work done.

Next, I'll give you my step-by-step guide to creating and implementing print assets that pre-sell your prospects. This includes shock-and-awe packages designed to wow your prospects by answering all their questions, handling their objectives, and enticing them to say yes to what you recommend. I'll teach you how to create a shock-and-awe package tailored to your practice and your unique message. You'll learn about the power of a case presentation package and how this asset can turn any employee into a master salesperson capable of educating and selling patients on your recommended treatment. Finally, we'll review unique and customizable print assets such as smile books, expertly crafted sales letters, welcome boxes, and many more—all designed to attract prospects, keep patients happy, and urge them to refer their friends and family to you for their dental concerns.

I'll also cover your digital power. Your website is your online storefront; it's not real estate, it's pixel estate—and your pixel estate can be one of your greatest strengths or weaknesses depending on the message it conveys and how it's designed. A clunky, outdated website that explains little is likely to turn potential patients away. You need a website, pixel estate, that attracts and persuades your ideal patients. This is done in a series of pages designed to educate and persuade. Your website should be a lead-capturing machine that lures prospects with excellent content they want and need to know.

We'll discuss how to drive patients to your website and encourage them to engage with you once there. We'll talk about how to make YouTube and social media ads perform, how to effectively use geofencing with marketing campaigns, and everything you need to know about search engine optimization (SEO) and organic and paid search campaigns.

No digital campaign would be complete without effective sales funnels and lead-capturing landing pages. We'll discuss the types of effective funnels that draw patients in and have them eagerly giving you their contact information to receive access to valuable content.

We'll also talk about long-term email campaigns and automated email sequences. These well-crafted assets will keep patients and prospects thinking of you and make them eager to refer their friends and family.

We will tie everything together and help you streamline your business with automation and management systems that save you time and money while ensuring your business runs according to your standards. You'll love how easy and effective these assets are to use and the magic they can add to your marketing efforts, client relationship management, and more.

Lastly, you're going to read some truly remarkable success stories. You'll hear from practice owners and dentists just like you who started hungry for growth and now own million-dollar and multi-million-dollar dental practices that attract a continuous flow of dental implants and high-end dental patients.

If you want to transform your practice, attract higher-value patients, work less, and earn more than ever, you are in the right place. If you know you need a marketing strategy that drives your ideal prospects to say yes to recommended treatment, you'll love what I have in store. If you've always wanted an automated direct response system that converts leads and keeps customers happy, you'll know exactly how to create this system and have it working like a well-oiled marketing machine by the time you finish this book.

So, without further delay, let's dive into developing your comprehensive growth strategy.

Chapter 1
Your Comprehensive Growth Strategy

Socrates said the first step toward wisdom is to know yourself.

I've often said achieving sustainable success is almost impossible if you don't know where you stand with your business.

When I first talk with dentists, most assume they understand their business. They think they know how their clients are handled and how leads are generated and harvested. They believe they have a good idea of who their high-value clients are. They assume they have a grasp on financial ratios tied to profitability, solvency and liquidity.

> *"A wise man investigates what others make assumptions about."*
>
> **- Jim Rogers**

I insist all my clients, whether they think they know their business or not, dive deep into their business.

The wise dentists I meet with never mind this. They understand the power of knowledge, often perform their own internal investigations, can quickly provide many of the answers, and gladly dive deep into their spreadsheets to find the rest.

I hope you're a wise dentist. I hope you recognize the value of fully understanding your strategy and analytics. I won't be able to insist you complete this step, but I'll tell you this: You will NEVER get all you can out of your time with this book if you simply skim over this chapter. You may make some money with a quick tip you pick up but if you're serious about building wealth, diving deep into your business and understanding where you stand is a crucial first step.

> *"Your current reality is the launching pad for your desired future. Embrace it, understand it, and then transcend it."*
>
> **- Robin Sharma**

Put the investigative tools I outline in this chapter to work to get a clear picture of the following aspects of your business economics:

- Cost per lead
- Cost per sale
- Current revenue versus your desired revenue
- The lifetime value of a new patient
- How many leads and sales you need to make up the difference
- Your value proposition regarding the problems your patients experience
- The hot-button issues that will get and hold a good prospect's attention and, often, get the desired response

So, dive deep with me. Gain a clear understanding so we can develop a road map, a strategic plan to optimize everything, and sell more implants and high-end dental services.

A deep dive involves identifying where you are today and what steps you need to install and implement a dental implant growth system in your practice.

I highly recommend using a mind-mapping program, but a piece of paper and a pen will do.

Your first step is to centralize your thoughts, planning elements, concepts, assumptions, beliefs, and the general principles at play within the framework of your business.

You need to identify choices and the overall results achieved to date.

This will act as a visual record and serve as a baseline for developing the plan that takes your business to new heights.

Use this mind-mapping session to identify your business goals, objectives, why you're in business, your personal and business history, previous failures and successes, priorities, and your wish list.

Once you've laid out these elements, it's time to perform a fundamental SWOT Analysis.

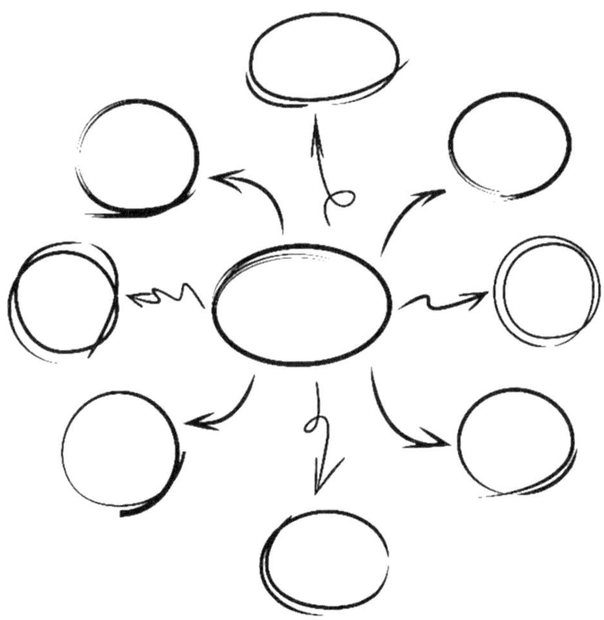

SWOT ANALYSIS: IDENTIFY, UNDERSTAND AND PREPARE

A SWOT analysis highlights your business's Strengths, Weaknesses, Opportunities and Threats. We take SWOT analysis one step further by identifying four core strategies:

1. **SO Strategy (Strengths-Opportunities):** You want to identify your strengths, such as your highly skilled and experienced dental staff, a modern and well-equipped dental clinic, strong patient relationships, or a good reputation in your community. Next, look at your opportunities. Maybe there's a growing demand for cosmetic dentistry in your area or an increasing population of older and affluent homeowners. By identifying these strengths and opportunities, you can develop a marketing campaign, maybe one that highlights the benefits of dental implants to an older individual and offers special promotions to attract new patients.
2. **WO Strategy (Weaknesses-Opportunities):** One weakness to address may be your limited online presence and previous failed marketing attempts. The opportunity may be excellent prospects you can find by exploring your database. In this scenario, the strategy may be developing educational content and implementing effective landing pages (more on this in chapters to come) that establish you as an authority on dental implants and presell your patients on the treatment you recommend.
3. **ST Strategy (Strengths-Threats):** This involves identifying internal strengths that can help counter external threats. Strengths such as strong patient relationships can help combat competition from nearby dental practices or economic downturns like we've all experienced over the past few years. One strategy may be considering loyalty programs or referral incentives to retain patients and attract new ones.
4. **WT Strategy (Weaknesses-Threats):** This helps address where you are most vulnerable by identifying your internal weaknesses and external threats. Your weaknesses may include a limited marketing budget or lack of ability to get patients to say yes to dental implants or expensive treatment. This can be compounded by increased competition from corporate dental chains and economic concerns that affect your patient's ability to pay. A strategy to address these types of threats could include making your marketing dollars count by creating persuasive messages and delivering them to a list of your ideal prospects. (All of which you can easily do with the strategies you're learning in this book.)

You must examine your business economics, including where you stand regarding total revenue, profit per transaction, your process for attracting new patients, your sales process once a new lead arrives, and the lifetime value of a new patient. You must analyze the treatment and services you offer and your value proposition, the hot-button issues that will get and hold your ideal prospects' attention and determine if these issues are covered in your current online and print assets.

By clearly understanding where you currently stand, you can decide where you want to be and what it will take to get there. This critical information helps develop your personal success blueprint that will guide your efforts and help you achieve steady, predictable growth and higher profits year after year.

The next step will help determine how much incremental growth you need quarter by quarter to reach your growth goal on schedule.

ASK YOURSELF THESE QUESTIONS:

1. What was last year's revenue?
2. What is your projected revenue for this year?
3. What percentage of current revenue is from implants?
4. How many locations do you have?
5. How many doctors?
6. How many owners?
7. How many family members as owners are in the practice?
8. What is your total number of patient files?
9. What type of dentistry is performed in your practice?
10. What is the total spending per year on online marketing?
11. What is the total spending per year on offline marketing?
12. How satisfied are you with your marketing?
13. What are the key practice elements you're looking to improve?

Next, it's time to ask yourself, "Where's the money?"

You need to understand the relationship between cost, volume and profit.

The goal is to gain a deep and robust understanding of how money, volume, cash flow, profit, and cost structure affect business choices, successes and failures, customer acquisition, retention tactics and strategies, and the need for change or course correction.

A Cost-Volume-Profit (CVP) Analysis will help you determine what you can cheerfully afford to spend to acquire a new client. This enables you to establish your risk tolerance and your ability to invest in testing various marketing methods, media and messages without breaking the bank.

TO PERFORM A CVP ANALYSIS:

1. Identify your variables and know your margins:
   - You need to know your sales price. How much do you charge for a single implant, a full-mouth restoration, gum therapy, and everything else?
   - What are your variable costs, including material, time and production?
   - What are your fixed costs for insurance, electricity and everything it takes to keep the doors open?
2. Know the difference between your cost and your sales price. *Contribution Margin = Sales Price per Unit - Cost per Unit*
3. Determine Your Break-Even Point:
   - The break-even point is the level of sales at which total revenue equals total costs, resulting in zero profit.
   - Break-Even Point (in units) = Fixed Costs / Contribution Margin
4. Analyze Your Profit at Different Levels of Activity:

   You can use the following formula:
   *Profit = (Sales Volume * Sales Price per Unit) - (Sales Volume * Variable Cost per Unit) - Fixed Costs*

A CVP analysis will help you make decisions about everything from pricing strategies to how many dollars you're willing to spend on marketing. And it will help you understand the risks and rewards associated with different offers and promotions. Please spend some time running these numbers. This will give you a great starting point and allow you to confidently decide everything from purchasing new operating systems to running a no-interest financing promotion.

Your next step is to analyze your current technologies: What roles do technology, web and data play in your practice?

Bill Gates often refers to technological processes, systems and databases as your digital nervous system. You must understand this system inside and out. What is the technological backbone of your practice? What databases are you currently using? What needs to be developed? How will it all work together?

YOU NEED TO EXAMINE:

- The role of technology in your practice.
- Your processes for handling online and offline data.
- The current state of technology components for your practice and the goals you have for the future.
- Your central marketing database system. Are you using HubSpot, GoHighLevel, ClickFunnels, Keap, Thryv, or other applications? We have developed our own proprietary system on the GoHighLevel platform, called eBGS: eLaunchers Best GROWTH System.
- Do you have old, stale or inaccurate data that needs to be updated with fresh, accurate and complete data?

All of these elements matter, and all must be evaluated to successfully move from where you are now to where you wish to be. Because the world of technology changes so rapidly, it's difficult to nail down one particular program or application in print. By the time you read this, there may be a better system in place than what's available as I write. I recommend doing your research, asking for recommendations, and ensuring your systems, databases, and technology are the right ones for your practice.

Part of your deep dive involves a hard look at all your marketing assets, including your message and offer.

Does your website look like it was purchased off the one-size-fits-all shelf?

Is it indistinguishable from competitors and littered with phrases such as "We value our clients," "We put you first," or "We've been serving our community for X years."

News flash: No one cares.

These statements are generic tripe most consumers ignore because they've heard it from people selling everything from toilets to roofing supplies to dental services.

If your marketing follows this cookie-cutter approach, it's causing you to lose patients.

You must be able to enter the conversation taking place in your prospect's head—the conversation that revolves around a problem they have or don't want to have and the result they want but don't have.

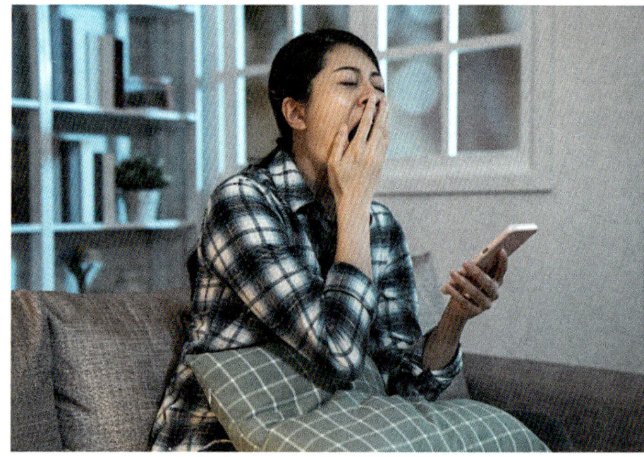

COMPETITIVE ANALYSIS: WHO IS DOING WHAT, TO WHOM?

Next, we must step outside your business and into your community to determine your biggest competitors and potential allies.

TAKE A LOOK AT YOUR COMPETITIVE POSITION IN YOUR MARKET. START BY ASKING THESE QUESTIONS:

- Who is your direct competition?
- Who is your indirect competition?
- Who can challenge or compete most effectively with you?
- Who can you most effectively compete with?
- Who has the "best clients" for your business currently?

You can learn a lot from your competition. Study what they're doing right and understand where they fall short. Read their reviews and discover what people love and hate about the services they offer. Learn from their failures and mistakes. Duplicate and expound on their success. Use your competition as a resource. They are targeting your market. Pay attention!

SYNERGISTIC/SYMBIOTIC RELATIONSHIPS AND JOINT VENTURES

It's not about resources but resourcefulness. Who in your industry and community will benefit from referring their trusted list of customers, clients, patients or patrons to you?

- Who can you partner with to access their customers?
- What relationships can you establish or grow to build your business?

- Whose client list is compatible with your goals?
- Who has the customers you want, and how can you collaborate with them?
- What businesses can you co-market with?

POTENTIAL SOURCES FOR THESE SYNERGISTIC RELATIONSHIPS INCLUDE:

General practitioners and family physicians. These medical professionals often have their patients' trust and can be an excellent referral source.

General dentists, periodontists, oral surgeons, or orthodontists who do not specialize in implant dentistry will gladly refer their patients to someone they trust and have a good relationship with.

Cosmetic surgeons have excellent lists of patients willing to pay for elective surgeries. A good relationship with a plastic surgeon can lead to referrals.

These are only a few examples that come to mind. The key is to think about your area and the professionals around you whose ideal customers, patients or patrons are similar to yours.

The key to your success is knowing where you are now, having a clear vision of where you wish to be, and understanding and implementing the steps necessary to get from one to the other. I hope you follow the steps in this chapter. If you do, you will be poised to experience growth at a level you may not have dreamed possible.

If you skimmed over this chapter or wish to continue reading before conducting your internal investigation, I urge you to return and spend some time here. From this point forward, we're hitting the ground running under the assumption you know exactly where your practice stands regarding the assets and systems we've discussed.

If you've done your research and now have a better understanding of where your practice stands today, then you'll love what I have in store for you in the next chapter. Stay tuned and discover the art of crafting a persuasive message that has your prospective patients lined up, cash in hand, eager for the smiles they've been dreaming of, and confident you are the go-to trusted source for dental implants.

Your Comprehensive Growth Strategy Workbook

This is the longest and most important end-of-chapter workbook. The information you gather in this section will be used throughout the rest of the book and in subsequent workbooks. Please spend some time on it because we are about to turn theory into application.

In this section, we will devise a comprehensive growth strategy for your practice.

Answer these questions and you will chart your course. Soon, you will have a map leading you toward a practice that consistently attracts your ideal, high-value patients.

YOUR GOALS AND OBJECTIVES

Setting clear goals and having defined objectives is crucial if you wish to build success.

What are your business goals?

Do you want to improve patient satisfaction and loyalty?
Expand your patient base?
Increase revenue?
Strengthen your online presence?
Develop a strong referral network with other health care professionals?
Implement effective marketing strategies to attract new patients?
Develop a positive and supportive work culture within your practice?
Achieve greater financial stability and growth?
Sell more dental implants and high-end cosmetic services?
Convert to a cash-only practice?
Bring in more associates?
Work fewer hours?
Increase the value of each patient?
Retain more referrals?
List your specific business goals here:

What are the specific objectives or measurable steps you will take to achieve your goals?

If your goal is to increase patient satisfaction and loyalty, then your objectives might be to:

- Implement patient feedback surveys to identify areas for improvement.
- Train staff members on excellent customer service techniques.
- Offer incentives for patient referrals and positive reviews.

If your goal is to expand your patient base and increase revenue, then your objectives might be to:

- Develop targeted marketing campaigns to attract new patients.
- Partner with local businesses and community organizations for outreach events.
- Offer flexible payment options and financing plans.

If your goal is to strengthen your online presence, then your objectives might be to:

- Optimize your website through the pixel estate strategies I outline in later chapters.
- Engage with patients on social media platforms.
- Have a long-term nurture campaign that offers valuable content to your patients and prospects.

If your goal is to implement effective marketing strategies to attract new patients, your objectives might be to:

- Conduct internal and market research to identify target demographics.
- Develop a comprehensive marketing plan, like the one outlined in this book, that includes online advertising, direct mail campaigns and community outreach.
- Track and analyze marketing metrics and evaluate the effectiveness of different strategies, then adjust as needed.

Once you clearly define your goals, list the key objectives, which are the measurable steps you will take to accomplish them.

"Failure is simply the opportunity to begin again, this time more intelligently." – Henry Ford

When designing your future, your past failures can be important indicators of what to avoid and what direction you should take.

What are your failures?

What are the moments in your career that you would rather not repeat?

- Did you launch expensive advertising campaigns that attracted the wrong types of patients, or worse, no patients?
- Have you neglected your online presence?
- Have you struggled with time management?
- Have you overworked yourself and neglected your own well-being?
- Have you hired a toxic staff member who interfered with daily operations and neglected customer service?

List your failures below. Be honest and specific. Writing them down will help you identify the mistakes you will not make again.

Now that you got that out of the way, it's time to toot your own horn a bit.

Workbook

What are your greatest successes so far in your practice?

- Do you have a great reputation with your patients?
- Are you an exceptional leader who can motivate, support and direct your staff?
- Do you have a firm grasp on money management and monitor spending with ease and efficiency?
- Do you have a particularly effective marketing strategy?
- Have you mastered asking for and receiving positive online reviews?

List your successes below. This will be your launching pad to achieve even greater success in the months and years to come.

We've discussed your goals, objectives, failures and successes. Now, let's talk about order and sequence.

What are your main priorities for the next six months? What about the next year? Five years?

- Do you want to grow your practice by attracting more high-value patients looking for dental implants and other cosmetic services?
- Would you like to get more value from the patient list you already have?
- Do you want to develop new relationships with general dentists and other health care professionals in your area to generate referrals?
- Are there parts of your practice's operational side that need improvement in terms of time management and customer service?

Think about the next several months, next year, and the next five years. What are your main priorities for your practice?

Now, let's talk about your wish list.

If you could wave your magic wand and have the practice of your dreams, what would it look like?

- Would you have a reputation in the community as an authority for all things dental? Would you be known as the trusted source for high-end cosmetic procedures?
- Would you have a cash-only practice brimming with patients who can easily afford your recommended treatment?
- Would you work less, maybe coming into the office only three or four days a week?

In this section, I want you to dream big. Let optimism be your guide and have fun. What is your dental practice wish list?

SWOT ANALYSIS

Your SWOT analysis will highlight your practice's Strengths, Weaknesses, Opportunities and Threats and help you to develop specific strategies to accomplish your goals.

What are your greatest strengths?

- Do you have a highly skilled and experienced dental team?
- A modern and well-equipped clinic?
- Strong patient relationships?
- A great reputation in your community?

List your greatest strengths below:

What are your weaknesses?

- Do you struggle with managing the financial end of your operation?
- Are you resistant to change?
- Do you micromanage your staff, fail to delegate and feel overworked?
- Is your website failing to attract new patients?
- Are your marketing techniques lacking?

Take a good hard look at your practice and management techniques and list the areas that need the most improvement:

That might have felt like a cold dose of reality, but by identifying your weaknesses, you also have identified opportunities for growth and improvement.
Identifying weaknesses is a great way to transition into opportunities for improvement.

What are your greatest opportunities?

- Is there a growing demand for cosmetic dentistry in your area?
- Is there an increase in older and affluent homeowners in the neighborhood?
- Are there general dentists and practitioners in your area you can partner with to gain referrals?
- Are there community outreach programs or networking opportunities you can access to help build your reputation in the community?
- Are there marketing strategies, like the ones outlined in this book, that you can use to get more value from your current patient list?

Spend a few moments thinking about the opportunities in your practice and your community, and list them here:

Now, let's discuss your biggest threats.

- What are the biggest hurdles you will need to overcome to achieve the level of success you dream of?
- Are there too many other practices competing for market share in your area?
- Is there an economic downturn in your community that makes it unlikely to attract high-end dental patients?
- Are your threats from within? Do you have toxic employees who routinely come in late, dampen morale, and fail to provide excellent patient service?

Spend some time with this and lay out the biggest external and internal threats to your success:

Once you have laid out your SWOT, review the section in this chapter on SWOT Analysis and consider which strategy will work best for you. By clearly understanding where you currently stand, you can decide where you want to be and what it will take to get there.

YOUR INCREMENTAL GROWTH CALCULATOR

The next step will help determine how much incremental growth you need quarter by quarter to reach your growth goal on schedule.

Ask yourself these questions:

- What was last year's revenue?
- What is your projected revenue for this year?
- What percentage of current revenue is from implants?

Workbook

- How many locations do you have?
- How many doctors are there at each location?
- How many owners do you work with?
- What is your total number of patient files?
- What type of dentistry is performed in your practice?
- What is the total spending per year on online marketing?
- What is the total spending per year on offline marketing?
- How satisfied are you with your marketing?
- What key practice elements are you looking to improve?

Once you have these answers, your next step is to perform a Cost-Volume-Profit Analysis.

Start by identifying your variables:

1. What are your sales prices? How much do you charge for single implants? Full-mouth restorations? Gum therapy? Hygiene? Everything else?

2. What are your variable costs, including material, time and production?

Now calculate the difference between your cost and your sales price.
Contribution margin = Sales price per unit – Cost per unit

Now, determine your Break-Even Point, or the level of sales at which total revenue equals total costs, resulting in zero profit.
Break-Even Point (in units) = Fixed Costs / Contribution Margin

Now that you have these metrics, you can analyze your profit at different levels of activity. You do this with the following formula:
*Profit = (Sales Volume * Sales Price per Unit) - (Sales Volume * Variable Cost per Unit) - Fixed Costs*

This Cost-Volume-Profit (CVP) Analysis will help you formulate pricing strategies, determine how much you're willing to spend on marketing, and understand the risks and rewards associated with different offers and promotions.
Now, it's time to perform a technology inventory.

WHAT ROLE DOES TECHNOLOGY PLAY IN YOUR PRACTICE?

- Do you have a website? Are you happy with it?
- Do you communicate with your current patients through text and email?
- Do you have long-term nurture strategies to keep in touch with current patients?
- Do you have outreach initiatives through social media?
- What processes do you currently have for handling online and offline data?
- What is your central marketing database system? Do you use HubSpot, GoHighLevel, ClickFunnels, Keap, Thryv, or other applications? We have developed our own proprietary system on the GoHighLevel platform, called eBGS: eLaunchers Best GROWTH System.
- What's the state of your data? Is it old, stale or inaccurate?

YOUR COMPETITIVE ANALYSIS: WHO ARE YOUR BIGGEST POTENTIAL ALLIES AND COMPETITORS?

- Who is your direct competition?
- Who is your indirect competition?
- Who can challenge or compete most effectively with you?
- Who can you most effectively compete with?
- Who has the "best clients" for your business currently?
- Who can you partner with to access their customers?
- What relationships can you establish or grow to build your business?
- Whose client list is compatible with your goals?
- Who has the customers you want and how can you collaborate with them?
- What businesses can you co-market with?

If you've spent time with this workbook, you now have a clear snapshot of where you are as a practice owner and where you wish to be. You have identified your greatest challenges and opportunities and outlined specific, actionable steps you can take to help you achieve your goals. The work you did in this section was time well spent and will help you implement the techniques and strategies in all the sections to come.

Chapter 2
The Magic of PRISM Research

Let's take a deep dive into your database.

As a data scientist, I have a superpower I'm about to share with you that will give you a tremendous advantage in your practice.

I NEVER guess WHO your ideal prospects are. I never guess why they buy. I never guess WHERE to find them. I dive deep into the data and discover who your best patients are, the ones who PAY, STAY and REFER.

Imagine the explosive growth you'd enjoy if every persuasive marketing message you send, online or off, reaches ideal candidates for dental implants and treatment. This is possible, and I will show you how PRISM research can help you identify your ideal prospects.

UNDERSTAND YOUR IDEAL PROSPECT WITH PRISM

PRISM Research gives you an unprecedented advantage in the marketplace. It allows you to reach out across your community with laser-like accuracy and identify the IDEAL people to benefit from dental implants and the high-end treatment you offer.

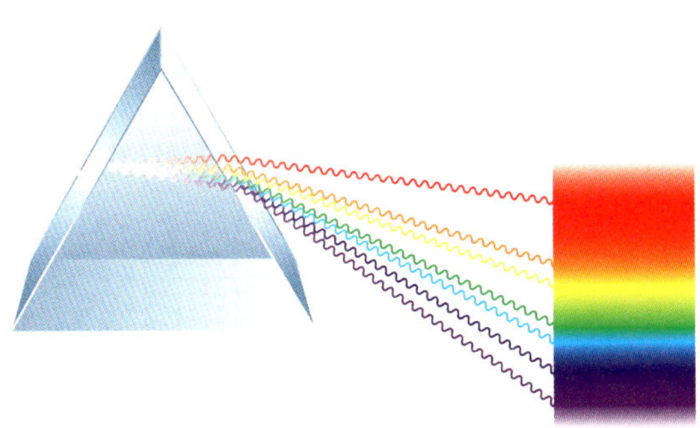

Just as a prism disperses light into its constituent colors, PRISM research disperses the information in your database into integral parts.

PRISM helps you identify the 20% of the patients responsible for 80% of your sales revenue. These are your best patients, the ones you wish they all were like.

With this information, you will create a data-driven avatar of precisely who your ideal prospects are.

This goes beyond the obvious.

When you're searching for your ideal customer in your database, you want to consider a variety of fields, including age, sex, income, homeowner, credit score, are they American Express card holders, stock market investors, their zip code, what magazine and newspaper subscriptions they hold, and more. The more detail, the better.

Now, it's doubtful you'll know the magazine subscriptions and stock preferences of your current client and prospect list. Still, this information is available with prestigious data sources, including MasterCard Analytics, D&B, Reference USA, Acxiom, Equifax, and others. The information you have in your database, paired with what you can gather from these sources, will help you understand your ideal prospects and, more importantly, create an avatar you can then market successfully to time and time again.

Dental Data Protocol helps you implement custom marketing campaigns that generate a robust stream of excellent prospects eager to say yes to dental implants or the treatment you recommend.

PRISM research helps you find unlimited prospects ideal for your practice and then effectively market to these prospects.

An essential part of PRISM is understanding how much your patients are worth to you—and yes, I'm speaking of a dollar amount. More specifically, what is the lifetime value of your patients?

You find this with a bit of quick, simple math. Take the average amount an average patient spends each year, including routine cleanings; multiply that number by the number of years a patient stays with you on average; then add the number of referrals sent. When you calculate this, you get the lifetime value of an average patient.

This number is specific to your practice and based on calculations only you can make, but knowing this number provides valuable insight into the type of dentistry you'll want to practice moving forward.

Most dentists recommend routine and basic cleanings once a year. These cleanings typically cost about $165 and usually take the dentist or hygienist 30 minutes to an hour to complete.

For a practice specializing in dental implants, a patient's average value starts at about $6,000.

These numbers tell us a general dentist will need SIX THOUSAND ordinary dental patients to equal the net revenue of 165 to 170 implant patients.

Considering there are only about 2,000 working hours a year, a dentist serious about grossing a million dollars in new net revenue cannot achieve this with general dentistry alone.

TO REACH EACH MILLION DOLLARS IN NET NEW REVENUE

FULL-MOUTH MAKEOVER @ $25,000	42 patients
SINGLE ARCH @ $12,000	84 patients
SINGLE TOOTH IMPLANT @ $6,000	167 patients
SINGLE REG. DDS. APPOINTMENT @ $165	6,000 patients!

The average dentist spends a fortune on different practice growth methods that fail to deliver results—seminars, coaching programs, websites, social media, magazine ads...I could go on.

Most dentists spend money on marketing and when they're disappointed with the results, they spend more money on marketing or change their marketing around to generate more leads.

Practice owners are often overwhelmed with their marketing and become victims of unfocused goals, unrealistic results for their current marketing, bad lists, and many other problems.

Is this you?

If you're in this group, you're not alone.

Many practice owners hesitate to try new marketing approaches, having been burned before with poor results. They spend so much time and money on ineffective marketing and start to believe all marketing efforts amount to no more than expensive wastes of time and resources. The result: 99% of dentists who spend money on marketing are unhappy with the results.

PRISM helps identify your ideal prospects who are ready to say yes now and those who are not quite ready to say yes but likely will be in the future.

Most marketing campaigns only go after low-hanging fruit—prospects ripe with interest. I call them Fit and Fast. They have a pressing need for dental services and may already have you in mind as their provider of choice.

Average marketing campaigns do little more than wave at these prospects. They say, "Why yes, we're here, we're still in business, and because you have a pressing need for dental services, let us help." I call this placeholder marketing because it amounts to little more than an "Open" sign in front of your physical building.

Marketing like this does nothing to attract potential patients who can benefit from dental implants or high-end dental services but are not quite ready to say yes, prospects I refer to as Fit and Slow. These men and women may be excellent candidates—with missing teeth, decaying teeth, or serious dental problems AND the financial resources necessary to fix these dental disasters. Still, for whatever reason, they haven't prioritized their problems. They are not yet ready to commit to treatment.

Ignoring this gold mine of potential patients is why most marketing efforts fall short. The MAJORITY of your prospects are in the "Fit and Slow" category. Eventually, they will buy, but only when they think they're ready.

You need three crucial elements to effectively market any product to anyone: The right list. The right message. The right product.

We'll dive into all three of these elements in the following chapters, but let's focus on building the right list for now.

> *"When your list is wrong…Nothing else matters!"*
> – Parthiv Shah

I've been building and selling mailing lists since 1989 and have mailed more than a BILLION pieces of direct mail.

In November 2022, I was awarded U.S. Patent# 11,507,967 for developing a business growth strategy based on data found in your QuickBooks. Bottom line, I KNOW LISTS.

Targeting the right audience or customer is essential. And you can identify those who belong on this list through PRISM research. PRISM identifies individuals or groups most likely to desire and need what you offer.

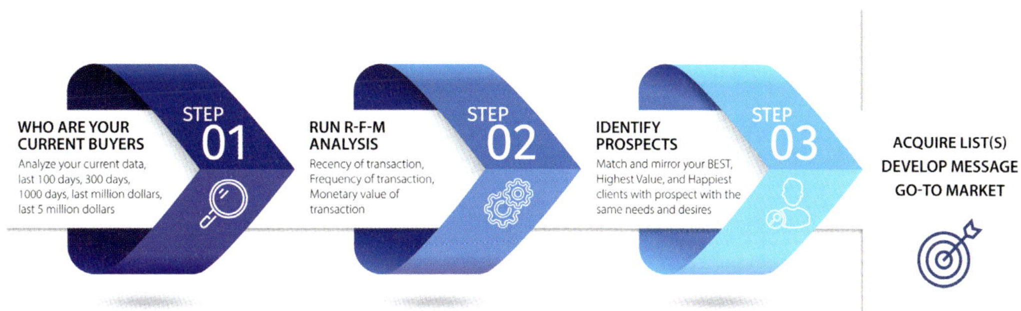
WHO ARE YOUR CURRENT BUYERS
Analyze your current data, last 100 days, 300 days, 1000 days, last million dollars, last 5 million dollars
STEP 01
RUN R-F-M ANALYSIS
Recency of transaction, Frequency of transaction, Monetary value of transaction
STEP 02
IDENTIFY PROSPECTS
Match and mirror your BEST, Highest Value, and Happiest clients with prospect with the same needs and desires
STEP 03
ACQUIRE LIST(S)
DEVELOP MESSAGE
GO-TO MARKET

PRISM is all about data-driven marketing.

You're about to learn to use data analysis and modeling to identify potential implant patients within your files. By analyzing patient data, you can pinpoint individuals likely to be interested in implant dentistry and create targeted marketing campaigns to reach them. This targeted approach allows you to maximize your marketing efforts and reach the right audience with the right message.

Dig for diamonds in your database.

Never use the marketing "hope" method of running advertising and "hoping" implant patients will call while ignoring the ones who already expressed interest. I recommend using Dan Kennedy's Renegade Millionaire System's 80/15/4/1 model to identify your current patients, who your past patients were, and which ones, the top 1% and 4%, are your highest value, most ideal patients. This process helps us identify where you want to go in pursuit of your next set of customers.

TO DO THIS, YOU MUST FOCUS ON:

- Identifying who your current buyers are.
- Running RFM Analysis: How **recent** are the transactions? What is the **frequency** of transactions? What's the **monetary** value of these transactions?
- What patterns, good or bad, can you glean from this analysis?
- Identify prospects. Match and mirror your BEST, highest value, and happiest clients with prospects with the same needs and desires.
- Optimization numbers: How effective are you, or not, relative to converting opportunities into sales, and what can you do to impact this equation favorably?

The best way to identify prospective high-value patients in your list is by using the patient-finding tools inside the commonly used Dental Intel software created by Dr. John Meise. If you're not using Dental Intel, I highly recommend you reconsider; I believe this to be one of the best tools available to assist dental practices. It has hundreds of applications. I'll highlight just one right now, but this one alone shows its worth. If, instead of Dental Intel, you're using an off-the-shelf software tool such as Patient Prism, Google Data Studio, or Databox, these will work for you, too.

Here's how it works.

I want you to run a report. Run ONE report in Dentel Intel (DI) that looks like this: Active patients aged 50 and over. They must have been seen within the last 24 months and paid more than $2,000 to your practice for dental services. Identify the patients who have unscheduled treatment of $2,000 or more but do not have an upcoming appointment. Run this report. It takes about a minute to build. For every million dollars you have in top-line revenue, you will find about 150 to 200 patients who meet these criteria. These are the diamonds in your database and where you can start an effective marketing campaign.

How Dental Intel made two practice owners millions by identifying diamonds in the Database.

A few years ago, I worked with a general practice owner with about $9 million in revenue and multiple dentists.

They did some implant work but wanted to do more.

I exported the patient database from Dental Intel and looked at the numbers.

They had 34,000 total patients, with 14,000 who accepted treatment and 19,000 who did not.

This equated to more than $145 million worth of unscheduled treatment.

This was an incredible, untapped opportunity.

By implementing the marketing system you'll learn about in the upcoming chapters, they converted a portion of these unscheduled cases into implant patients.

We used this data to develop tailor-made digital and direct mail marketing campaigns. The results were phenomenal, with an influx of high-end patients, the likes of which the practice had never experienced before.

Here's another example. This dental client had three locations and about $8 million in top-line revenue. I dove into his practice software, and in less than three minutes, I generated a report identifying 472 leads that could result in $2.1 million in revenue if we targeted them with a specific campaign.

I developed the list with the following criteria: Patients over age 50 who had been in for treatment in the past two years and had made cash payments for this treatment; had been given a non-insurance treatment plan valued at more than $2,000; had declined that treatment and currently did not have an appointment scheduled. Next, we created online and offline marketing campaigns similar to the ones I'll review in detail in future chapters. The targeted campaigns were a huge success, resulting in a surge

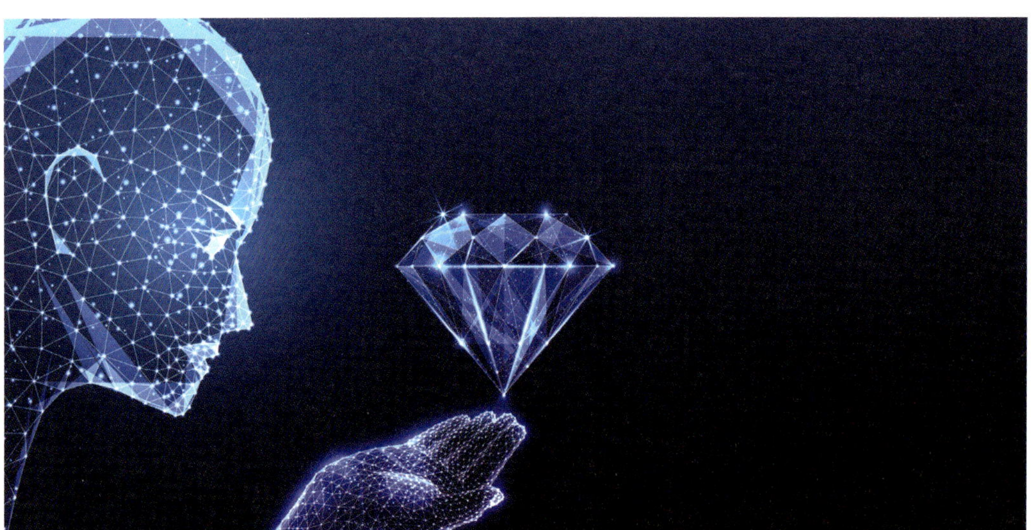

of high-value dental implant patients eagerly agreeing to treatment.

These are just two examples. I have a 35-year career filled with similar successful marketing campaigns.

Are diamonds slipping through your fingertips?

For every new patient, you likely lose between six and 12 who did not convert. Some never call in the first place, some don't attend their appointments, and others come in only to decline treatment.

This happens because most practices have no follow-up marketing efforts for potential patients who did not instantly agree to treatment. Without the proper follow-up, these $6,000 leads simply walk away.

Part of your Dental Data Protocol involves an in-depth analysis of your last three months, 12 months, and three years of revenue data. This way, we can spot trends of WHO buys, WHAT they buy, and WHY they buy. We can see who is NOT buying and WHY they said no to treatment.

Every patient is precious, but some are more precious than others. This data analysis aims to identify HOT pockets of opportunities we can strike at with whatever marketing budget you have.

In the chapters to come, we will discuss the importance of nurturing leads, educating patients and showing them why agreeing to dental implants with your clinic is in their best interest. For now, I want you to see the potential power of a good list that might just be a few clicks away.

In the next chapter, we'll take PRISM Research to the next level and dive even deeper into Dental Data Protocol. You'll soon know the exact steps you'll need to take to identify your ideal prospects in your internal database and acquire external lists of ideal patients already eager for your marketing message.

The Magic of PRISM Research Workbook

PRISM research is all about taking a deep dive into your database and coming out with valuable insight into how to reach out and connect with your ideal patients.

You'll want to spend some time with this workbook because what you discover could easily increase your revenue by 20% to 50% or more.

Let's start with a series of questions:

Who are your ideal prospects? Are they male or female? Young or old? Do they own their own homes? Do they have American Express Cards?

The key to PRISM research is identifying the 20% of patients responsible for 80% of your sales revenue.

Take a few moments to describe the types of patients you most want to attract to your practice:

By identifying your ideal prospects and the patients responsible for the lion's share of your sales revenue, you can design and implement custom marketing campaigns that generate a robust stream of excellent prospects eager to do business with you.

An essential part of PRISM is understanding how much your patients are worth to you—and yes, I'm speaking of a dollar amount. More specifically, what is their lifetime value?

You find this with a bit of quick, simple math.

Take the average amount an average patient spends each year, including routine cleanings. Multiply that by the average number of years they stay with you and add the number of referrals they send. When you calculate this, you get the lifetime value of an average patient.

This number is specific to your practice and based on calculations only you can make. Knowing it provides valuable insight into the type of dentistry you'll want to practice from this point forward.

Most dentists recommend routine and basic cleanings once a year. These cleanings typically cost about $165 and usually take the dentist or hygienist 30 minutes to an hour to complete.

For a practice specializing in dental implants, a patient's average value starts at about $6,000.

These numbers tell us a general dentist will need SIX THOUSAND ordinary dental patients to equal the net revenue of 165 to 170 implant patients. Once you've decided who your ideal patients are and what type of patients you wish to attract, you can design a custom-made marketing campaign to attract more of them to your practice.

A crucial element of having an effective marketing campaign is having the right list.

PRISM is all about data-driven marketing and finding diamonds in your database.

Use the list below to identify prospective high-value patients in your database. Once you have the metrics you wish to use, you can run a report with the patient-finder tools inside the Dental Intel software.

1. Identify who your current buyers are.
2. Run RFM Analysis: How recent are the transactions? What is their frequency? What's their monetary value?
3. What patterns, good or bad, can you glean from this analysis?
4. Identify prospects. Match and mirror your BEST, highest value, and happiest clients with prospects who have the same needs and desires.
5. Determine optimization numbers: How effective are you at converting opportunities into sales, and what can you do to improve this equation?

If you've spent time with this workbook, you have a clear understanding of who your ideal patients are and which patients are currently generating the greatest income for your practice. You've searched your database with the criteria indicated and should have a list of ideal candidates for dental treatment.

With this information, you are ready to move on to phase two of this process: Dental Data Protocol.

Chapter 3
Dental Data Protocol: Find and Collect Your Diamonds

In the previous chapter, we discussed PRISM Research and how this powerful tool can help you comb through your own database and methodically identify your ideal prospective patients and compile a list of excellent candidates for high-end dental treatment and dental implants.

In this chapter, we take it a step further. I'll discuss the steps necessary to find these diamonds in your own database or through external sources to compile a list of ideal prospective patients. Dental Data Protocol is about finding and collecting your diamonds.

First, let's start with your internal lists.

If you're familiar with the book by Russell Conwell, *Acres of Diamonds*, you know the story about the man who sold his family farm to search for diamonds, never realizing the land he left behind was rich with them. The story is meant to be a cautionary tale, a warning, and a bit of sage advice all wrapped into one. The idea is that before you seek your fortune elsewhere, you should first look within. If you've been in business for any number of years and achieved even moderate success, you likely have a database brimming with undiscovered diamonds. Dental Data Protocol is about helping you find and collect these diamonds, these ideal patients with a desperate need for dental implants and the ability to say yes to the treatment you recommend.

As a dentist, you have a unique set of challenges and opportunities. You spend money on social media, search engine optimization (SEO), direct mail advertising, advertising events, and increasing word of mouth. Most of these efforts give you at least some results. You generate a lot of leads, and a fraction of these leads turn into new patients.

Here's how it might work:

You decide to run a dental implant marketing campaign and commit $10,000 in cash or human energy, effort and time. Whether you focus on online efforts with SEO or offline efforts with direct mail or marketing events, it doesn't matter. If the campaign is at least moderately successful, your $10,000 will generate about 200 leads. Out of those 200 leads, about 20 will actually call and set an appointment. Out of the 20 who set an appointment, 16 will actually show up. Twelve of the 16 who show up will be qualified to buy, and 10 of those will say yes to implants and follow through with treatment. This formula is predictable and profitable. It happens time and time again with slight variation and keeps most dentists happy.

It's easy to understand why. You spend $10,000 on marketing efforts that attracts 10 new implant or high-end dentistry patients to your office. The average fee collected for dental implants, cosmetic procedures, and sedation dentistry is about $6,000. That means for your $10,000 investment, you collect $60,000. Not bad at all. You're happy, and you should be.

The problem is, for every 10 patients you sell, you have 190 leads that can be categorized as either good leads, bad leads, unscheduled treatments, lost opportunities, or unconverted leads that you, and almost every other dental practice in the industry, will likely not thoroughly pursue. This diamond mine of unconverted lead and lost opportunity is usually neglected and ignored.

If you're really on top of things, you may make a few phone calls, possibly send out an email follow-up or text, but then, in 20 days or less, that's it—those leads go to your mental trash can, never to be thought of again.

During all my years consulting with dental practice owners, I've found most are guilty of neglecting the diamonds in their database. So, if you are guilty of this, you are not alone, and I point this out not to chastise you but to highlight an opportunity.

It's easy to understand why you'd abandon prospective patients who did not instantly agree to treatment. You're a dentist. You're busy. You spend your time treating and caring for the patients who say yes. You may not feel like you have time to chase down all the naysayers. And this is true, you don't have time for that. You need systems in place that do the heavy lifting for you, that educate, indoctrinate, and nurture these prospective patients.

You need an extended follow-up system that acts as a dental practice growth machine by helping you stay in touch with your prospects. You need to educate them, indoctrinate them, and nurture them about implants, treatment, and the transformation they can expect in their lives once they say yes to treatment.

Dentists have a unique set of problems when helping patients. When people suffer a heart attack and are told to see a cardiologist, they go. They don't put it off, thinking their money or time would be better spent on a car or remodeling a bathroom. If they develop a strange spot on their nose and discover they have skin cancer, they don't say, "That can wait till later," and go on about their business. They see an oncologist immediately because they understand these problems threaten everything. Their LIFE is in jeopardy.

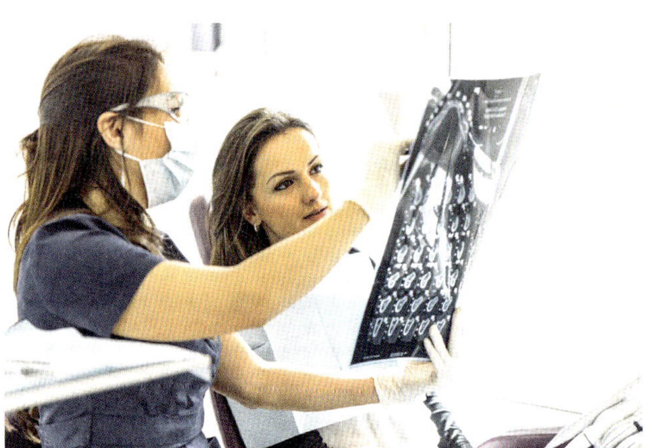

Most people, unless they're in pain, do not associate a sense of urgency with dental problems. They don't understand what's at risk with a missing or decayed tooth, bleeding gums, or an unchecked toothache. Most patients have no clue there's an oral-systemic connection between periodontal disease, cardiovascular disease and organ failure. They see their teeth and oral health almost as a separate system and a missing tooth as nothing more than a cosmetic blemish or mild inconvenience.

This is why, as a dentist, you must educate your patients on the negative consequences associated with dental neglect. You have an obligation to educate them and help them understand what's at stake if they neglect their oral health and just live with a mouth full of rotten or missing teeth.

If your patients don't own their disease—if they don't understand their teeth, jawbone, appearance, self-esteem, and even their life are at risk by failing to address their oral health concerns— they will often choose to do nothing. They need to be motivated to solve their problems and solve them now.

They need to see a missing tooth as an incapacitating ailment, just like a missing limb. Without their teeth, they can't chew, bite or smile confidently—all three necessary activities in human living.

Patients need to understand how implant dentistry protects the integrity of their jawline, safeguards them from harmful bacteria, and adds life to their years with a renewed ability to laugh, smile and chew the foods they love.

They need to understand all of these things, and it's up to you to educate them.

The last problem is most insurance plans, under most circumstances, will not pay for implant or cosmetic dentistry. This gives prospective implant patients the idea that because it's not covered by insurance, it must not be necessary or all that important. If it were, surely insurance would pay for it. You know this is nonsense. I know it's nonsense. Still, the majority of your patients simply do not understand.

The unique nature of dentistry creates a unique set of challenges, no doubt. But with these challenges come opportunities.

Because of these challenges, there are more diamonds in your database than if you were a general doctor or a physician—and it's why you need systems in place to help you connect with, educate, indoctrinate, and nurture your prospects. These systems are easy to use once you understand how, and I will go into this in great detail in chapters to come. But for now, let's just say effective marketing efforts aimed at these diamonds in your database can be a game changer in your practice.

So, now you have an idea of the untapped potential in your practice. You're likely thinking about past marketing campaigns or lists of patients with unaccepted or unscheduled treatment. Now, let's turn our focus to gathering information on prospective patients and compiling a dynamic list of ideal dental implant candidates.

STEP 1: CONNECT YOUR PRACTICE MANAGEMENT SYSTEM TO MARKETING AUTOMATION

Assuming you have a practice management system such as Dentrix, Eaglesoft or Open Dental, you will want to connect with a dashboard tool. I highly recommend Dental Intelligence (Dental Intel) for its simplicity and the wide range of tools and features it offers to help with data analytics and patient communications.

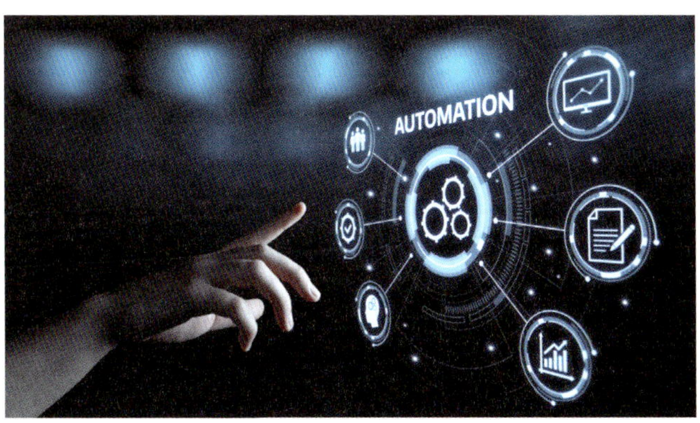

If you don't have a practice management system that integrates with Dental Intel, you can still do all the things I recommend in this chapter; it will just be more difficult for you. If your practice management system connects to something else, you can create a custom integration to extract data from your practice management system and push it to your marketing automation system, or you can assign a human in your office to export reports daily or weekly to push the data in your marketing automation system.

Think of it like a GPS: the No. 1 rule is not only to have a clear understanding of where you want to go but to have an even clearer understanding of where you are right now. You have to know where you are now and where you wish to go to build a road map. As it relates to your data, you must understand your geography and your demographics to know how to direct your marketing efforts and how you wish to market to your ideal prospects.

Once again, this is why I recommend Dental Intel. You need a platform that helps with data analytics, Key Performance Indicator (KPI) tracking, patient communication, appointment scheduling, practice management and integration. Dental Intel does all of this.

This may seem like a sales pitch, but I want you to understand the power of this platform. And if you're using something similar, you'll see the power in what you use as well.

DENTAL INTEL:

- Helps you analyze performance data while offering insights and actionable information to improve operations, scheduling and patient care.
- Helps track KPIs to monitor and optimize aspects of your practice, such as patient retention and case acceptance.
- Boosts patient communications with tools to improve patient engagement, appointment scheduling and follow-up.
- Provides practice management tools to help manage patient records and improve your practice's efficiency and flow.

Whether you use Dental Intel or something else, you need to analyze your data to determine the avatar for your ideal patient. Complete list research to identify potential prospects for dental implants based on specific criteria and characteristics. This includes demographic information, behavioral data, age, gender, and other socioeconomic factors. This information will help you identify your ideal patient.

Clearly identifying your ideal prospects from your internal lists also will help you with external acquisition from list brokers or with targeted ads on social media.

Dental Intel software has a tool called Patient Finder that allows you to run custom searches on actual patient data (active and inactive) and create segmented lists based on criteria selected by you or your marketing agency trained in Dental Intel. Here is an example report:

Active patients who have been seen by the practice within the last two years, age 50 + , and who have unscheduled treatment of more than $2,000 with treatment code IMPLANT will give you a list of your implant diamonds in your database.

Here are some additional reports you can run from your practice management system:

- Inactive patients
- Active patients
- Patients over 50 with an email address
- Patients over 50 without an email address
- Patients with Blue Cross Blue Shield PPO as their medical insurance provider
- Patients without insurance (so we can market your in-office dental care plan to them)
- Patients with no-recall (so we can run reactivation campaigns)

Once we have the reports, you can read the data and create a unique strategy for each market segment. With the information you get from these reports, not only do you know who your ideal patients are, but you know a lot about them. This means you will be able to craft a marketing message that resonates because you'll have a better understanding of who they are and what concerns them.

STEP 2: GATHER YOUR DATA SO YOU KNOW EXACTLY WHAT'S HAPPENING TO YOUR LEADS

What are you doing to schedule appointments?

- What happens when an incoming call comes into your office?
- What happens when someone fills out a form?
- What happens to leads generated by social media?
- Do you run referral contests? What happens to that data?
- Do you get referrals from other general practice centers?
- Do you get referrals from physicians?
- Do you do any event marketing? Where do you house all the leads?
- What about appointment no-show patients who book appointments and do not show up? These no-shows are your inactive patients who meet your criteria.
- Who are your inactive patients with Blue Cross Blue Shield for their medical insurance?
- What about appointment no-sales?
- How about active and inactive patients with missing teeth who took a case presentation but did not buy? You can get this from your practice management or system report or by using Dental Intel's Patient Finder.

Knowing what's happening to your leads will help compile your list of prospects and organize your processes. If you are NOT capturing this data, you have a systemic data loss that needs to be fixed before you can move forward.

STEP 3: GET A DATABOX ACCOUNT

You can buy your own at databox.com and set up your own dashboard. The purpose of your Databox dashboard will be to track activities from five data points:

- Google My Business for Google Local Listing
- Google Analytics for Organic Search Volume
- Google Ads for Google Pay Per Click Campaigns
- Facebook Pages for your organic activities on social media
- Facebook Ads for your Facebook paid advertising campaigns

Tracking these activities provides valuable insights into the performance of your online marketing efforts. This lets you assess their effectiveness and understand how various channels contribute to your success.

By monitoring online activities and their associated metrics, you can determine your ROI for specific marketing campaigns. This will help you allocate resources efficiently and make data-driven decisions regarding your marketing budget.

Most importantly, tracking these activities will help you understand your target audience's demographics, behaviors and preferences. This information is crucial for tailoring marketing campaigns to specific patient segments and improving your chances of reaching your ideal patients.

Depending on your current digital marketing strategies and vendors, you may need additional dashboards to track your spending and the outcome.

If you can't measure it, you can't manage it.

Now that you've identified your internal lists and are tracking your external marketing efforts, you need to identify what's working and what's not. How? One of the best ways is through dedicated tracking numbers that ring to your business.

The tool I use for my clients is CallPro, available through MVP. You can learn more about this at www.tinyel.com/callpro. With CallPro, you can have dedicated tracking numbers that ring to your main business phone number. They can be added to whatever you want tracked. We typically assign individual tracking numbers to these traffic sources:

1. Website
2. Email marketing automation campaigns, funnels and print assets
3. No set marketing campaigns
4. No-show marketing campaigns
5. No-sell marketing campaigns
6. One extra number to be used for other campaigns

You can buy as many phone numbers as needed to track lead sources of incoming phone calls. Then, CallPro helps monitor what happens when someone calls you from one of these sources.

The call is recorded. Missed call alerts are automatically sent to you so you can call back. Then, CallPro reviews the calls and scores them by MVP's Call Quality Analysts. Each call is scored on 20+ KPIs to grade your staff's effectiveness on the call and call outcome.

The cool part is you can track all of this on your personal CallPro dashboard. This lets you see the results of your marketing efforts and your staff performance. You also can listen to recorded calls.

This tool is powerful, not just for gauging marketing efforts but for assessing staff performance and determining if there may be a need for internal sales and customer service training.

Digital Marketing Traffic and Leads Reports

Depending on which digital marketing vendor you choose to work with, they will likely provide you with a dashboard or at least a self-populating Google Sheet with new leads generated by your online marketer when they spend money on paid traffic or make an effort to generate organic leads.

You should take those leads and bump them through external databases to "skip trace" the leads and gather the prospect's physical address. You can do this through credit reporting agencies, such as Equifax or TransUnion, or public record databases including searches for real estate purchases and property records.

The prospect's physical address will give you more intelligence about the dwelling type (single family versus condo versus townhome versus multi-family), home ownership, length or residence, mortgage, home equity, and other financial qualification/disqualification criteria like bankruptcy flag, judgment flag or lien flag.

The purpose of this additional data search is to identify qualified prospects from the leads generated by your digital marketers and add them to an offline direct mail marketing routine.

When you combine the lead data and contact information captured by Facebook, which tells you what your prospects are interested in, and Google, which tells you what they're searching for, with the corresponding housing data that tells you what they can afford, you get a powerful list of interested prospects who are actively seeking out what you provide and are likely able to afford to say yes to implants and the treatment you recommend.

Geographic/Demographic Heatmaps: Find Prospective Patients and Directly Market to Their Neighbors

Geographic/demographic heat maps are about identifying where your patients are located and directing marketing campaigns at their neighbors—the ones that look like them, live in similar houses, and can afford your services.

From your own database or from skip traces you perform on your Google and Facebook analytics, you can determine where your prospects live. This can help you decide which neighborhoods you wish to target with direct mail campaigns and allows you to get even more specific with geofencing with Facebook and Google ads.

When you export your patient database of active and inactive patients, you can pin them on the map to identify which zip codes, neighborhoods, and streets you are pulling patients from, run demographics/psychographics analysis (age, income, home value, presence of child/children and other parameters) and identify a database of neighbors. For a practice with a million dollars in current revenue, you will probably have 1,500 active patients and 3,500 inactive patients, so you should be able to get 25,000 to 50,000 neighbors who match and mirror the profile of your current patients.

Once you have the neighborhood data, you can give it to your Google and Facebook vendors to build a tighter geofence around zip codes and neighborhoods so you don't waste advertising dollars marketing outside your primary geographic market.

The database of neighbors is used to create your direct mail campaigns. Our preferred vendor, MVPMailhouse.com, currently sends out 5,000 postcards for $3,100. After mailing more than 100,000,000 postcards in dentistry, they have the postcard creation game down cold. You can use MVP Mailhouse or another postcard company to run a similar data-gathering process.

List Research and External Data Acquisition

Depending on what services you want to promote, you can identify geographic and demographic parameters and buy direct mail lists, telemarketing lists, and email marketing lists. Your offer helps you determine your segments, your segment helps you determine your offer, your offer helps you determine your marketing vehicle, and your marketing vehicle helps you determine your messages on the vehicle.

For example, with Facebook Ads, you can have no more than 125 characters with a headline of up to 40 characters and a link description of up to 30 characters. With a direct mail postcard, you can have about 70 words, and with a direct mail sales letter you can have as many as you'd like, with an average of about 5,000.

STEP 4: DATA MODELING

CAUTION: Only use this if you already have your ideal patients in your database. Skip this step if you're just getting started with dental implants and have been a general dentist up to this point without a list of implant patients in your database. Data modeling only applies if you already have some success with dental implants or high-end dental services.

If you have an internal list of ideal prospective patients, you can send this list to a database modeling provider such as Equifax or Acxiom.

When you send your current patient data for data modeling, the database modeling provider will append 1,000 to 1,500 columns to your patient database, craft a model of your current patient database's profile, and tell you how much market share of these patients you have captured in your selected geography. You can use the model data to buy a direct mail list of your prospective patients.

This is a very advanced, highly sophisticated technique that is used only when appropriate. If you are unhappy with WHO your current patients are, cloning them does not make sense. If you market to anyone and everyone, your current patient database will not have meaningful segmentation. Sometimes, the model makes inappropriate assumptions and may steer you in the wrong direction.

There are two types of errors in data modeling that we need to be careful about: Type 1 errors that add inappropriate prospects to your marketing list, resulting in wasteful marketing spending, and Type 2 errors that remove prospects who are highly likely to buy from you from your marketing list... and this has an opportunity cost.

Data modeling is not appropriate for every dental practice, and it should be done by trained data scientists with significant experience in direct mail data modeling and a reasonable understanding of how standard direct mail data modeling principles apply to your practice.

Data modeling is a potent technique used for due diligence and research when you're acquiring a current practice. When you are ready to buy someone's practice, have them connect their practice management system to a dashboard like Dental Intel and run various reports through Patient Finder. The exported patient database(s), active and inactive, should go through postal heat maps and demographic data modeling so you can read more about the patient database you are about to buy.

This sums up Dental Data Protocol. I hope you can see how this powerful tool will help you identify and compile a dynamic list of ideal patients who need and can easily afford high-end dentistry and dental implants.

Now comes the fun part. In the next chapter, you'll learn how to craft a marketing message that reaches into your ideal prospects' heads, educates them, indoctrinates them, and has them racing past your competitors, cash in hand, eager to accept the treatment you recommend and enjoy the life-changing benefits dental implants provide.

Workbook

Dental Data Protocol Workbook

How to find and collect diamonds in your database.

STEP 1: CONNECT YOUR PRACTICE MANAGEMENT SYSTEM TO MARKETING AUTOMATION

Whether you use Dental Intel Eaglesoft or Dentrix, you will need to connect your practice management system to a dashboard tool. I recommend Dental Intel. Dental Intel software has a tool called Patient Finder that allows you to run custom searches on your actual patient data (active and inactive) and create segmented lists based on criteria selected by you or your marketing agency trained in Dental Intel. Here is an example report:
Active patients who have been seen in your practice within the last two years, age 50 +, who have unscheduled treatment of more than $2,000 with treatment code IMPLANT will give you a list of your implant diamond patients already in your database.

Here are some additional reports you can run from your practice management system:

- Inactive patients
- Active patients
- Patients over 50 with an email address
- Patients over 50 without an email address
- Patients with Blue Cross Blue Shield PPO as their medical insurance provider
- Patients without insurance (so we can market your in-office dental care plan to them)
- Patients with no-recall (so we can run reactivation campaigns)

STEP 2: GATHER YOUR DATA SO YOU KNOW EXACTLY WHAT'S HAPPENING TO YOUR LEADS

What are you doing to schedule appointments?

- What happens when an incoming call comes into your office?

- What happens when someone fills out a form?

- What happens to leads generated by social media?

- Do you run referral contests? What happens to that data?

- Do you get referrals from other general practice centers?

- Do you get referrals from physicians?

- Do you do any event marketing? Where do you house all the leads?

- What about appointment no-show patients who book appointments and do not show up? These no-shows are your inactive patients who meet your criteria.

- Who are your inactive patients with Blue Cross Blue Shield for their medical insurance?

- What about appointment no-sales?

- How about active and inactive patients with missing teeth who took a case presentation but did not buy? You can get this from your practice management, system reports or by using Dental Intel's Patient Finder.

STEP 3: GET A DATABOX ACCOUNT

You can buy your own at databox.com and set up your own dashboard. The purpose of your Databox dashboard will be to track activities from five data points:

- Google My Business for Google Local Listing
- Google Analytics for Organic Search Volume
- Google Ads for Google Pay Per Click Campaigns
- Facebook Pages for your organic activities on social media
- Facebook Ads for your Facebook paid advertising campaigns

Workbook

Track your results.

How? One of the best ways to track advertising success is to use dedicated tracking numbers specific to your business.

There are several call tracking tools available on the market. While vendors or agencies might provide their own call tracking systems with campaign-specific phone numbers, it is a better idea to have your OWN phone tree. This way, you can track your own results and move phone numbers from one vendor to another whenever you choose to switch. With Call tracking tools, you can have dedicated tracking numbers that ring to your main business phone number. They can be added to whatever you want tracked. We typically assign individual tracking numbers to these traffic sources:

1. Website
2. Email marketing automation campaigns, funnels and print assets
3. No set marketing campaigns
4. No-show marketing campaigns
5. No sell marketing campaigns
6. One extra number to be used for other campaigns

Take the leads generated by your online marketing and bump them through external databases, such as credit reporting agencies, to capture their physical address.

The combination of patient demographic information, interests and hobbies, as identified by their Facebook activities and Google searches, helps you identify ideal prospects.

From your own database or from skip traces you perform on your Google and Facebook analytics, you can find where your prospects live. This can help you decide which neighborhoods to target with direct mail campaigns. It also allows you to get even more specific with geofencing with Facebook and Google ads.

Once you have the neighborhood data, your Google and Facebook vendors can build a tighter geofence around the zip codes and neighborhoods so you don't waste advertising dollars marketing outside your primary geographic market.

The database of neighbors is used to create your direct mail campaigns. Our preferred vendor, MVPMailhouse.com, currently sends out 5,000 postcards for $3,100. After mailing more than 100,000,000 postcards in dentistry, they have the postcard creation game down cold. You can use MVP Mailhouse or another postcard company, such as Upswell Marketing or Practice ZEBRA, to run a similar data-gathering process.

If you've spent time with this workbook, you understand the steps necessary to find the diamonds in your database. Combining what you discovered in the last chapter on PRISM Research and this chapter on Dental Data Protocol, you can now develop a spectacular list of potential, high-value dental patients who will likely say yes to the treatment you recommend. With this information, you're ready to move on to the next step: Crafting a marketing message that connects!

Chapter 4
Message to Market Matters

Successful dental practices thrive by drawing in droves of patients who need and can pay for dental implants, All-on-4s and other high-priced dental services. In this chapter, we'll discuss how to successfully identify your ideal high-value patients. Then, we'll talk about how to craft your marketing message in a way that has them speeding past your competitors, cash in hand, eager to do business with you. Match the right message to the right market and expect a surge of business from high-value patients who will have your practice brimming with business—scheduled weeks and months in advance.

If you followed my advice in the last chapter and dove deep into your business with the Dental Data Protocol, you are in a powerful place right now. You likely understand your business on a new level. You may have already identified the diamonds in your database by running reports through Dental Intel.

If you did, you're off to a great start and have taken the essential first steps to transform your practice into a dental implant-fueled profit-making machine.

If you spent some time with Dental Data Protocol, you're ready for the next step. This is where the magic happens. Now, it's time to craft a message that connects with your ideal patients—the ones you love doing business with and who will benefit from dental implants and the treatment you recommend, can easily afford to say yes, and are a pleasure to work with.

I want to start this discussion with a lesson from marketing genius Dan Kennedy.

During mastermind coaching sessions, Dan repeatedly emphasizes that in any population of people, including prospects ideal for dental implants, 1% are rich, 4% are affluent, 15% are price-sensitive buyers with little disposable income, and 80% are on edge financially and have no disposable income.

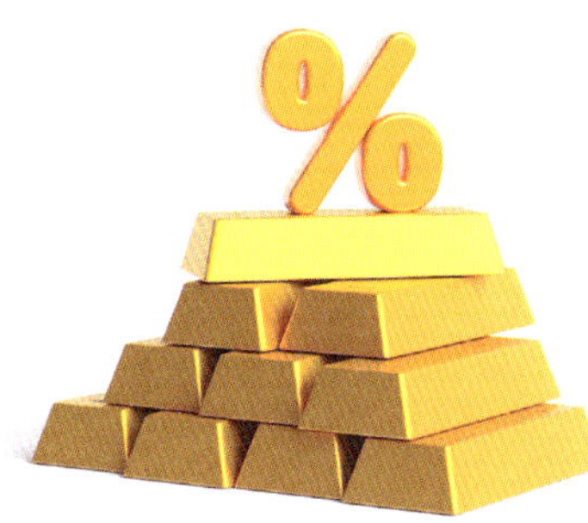

Your best prospects, the ones who will move the needle for you the fastest and make the biggest difference to your bottom line, are the high-value prospects, the top 5% of your pyramid of possible buyers.

The following 15% are so price-sensitive that making a sale is far more difficult. And the bottom 80% of this universe of potential patients can't afford to say yes, no matter how much they may wish to. Wasting marketing dollars on the bottom 80% equates to digging a hole, throwing your money inside, setting it on fire, and burying the ashes.

Smart business owners are happy to spend more to attract HIGH-VALUE PROSPECTS than they spend to attract average prospects who are more difficult to sell and will never be as likely to say yes to treatment as your top 5% high-value prospects.

Dan says one of the biggest mistakes business owners make, a mistake that keeps them from achieving a highly profitable business and has many barely getting by, is failing to identify and aggressively pursue this top 5% of high-value patient pyramid.

So, how do you identify the top 5%?

ASK YOURSELF:

- Who are your best patients?
- Who are the easiest to deal with?
- Who spent the most?
- Who were the quickest to agree to treatment?

By identifying your ideal patients, you craft an avatar of your ideal prospect, the one you wish to attract and want to do business with, as opposed to those who spend half as much and are twice as difficult to deal with.

Start by digging for diamonds in your database. Your current patient list is responsible for the success you've achieved so far, so dig in and do your research.

If you ran the internal reports I talked about in the last chapter, then you may already have an excellent list in your hands. Suppose you wish to look outside your business to find dental gems. In that case, I recommend speaking with a good list broker. Look for one who collects and curates lists of men and women who fit a profile similar to your ideal prospects...something like this:

- Homeowners in specific zip codes
- Over 50
- Who search online for terms like cosmetic dentistry and dental implants
- Who show similar interest in esthetics and maintaining a healthy lifestyle
- Possibly American Express Card Holders
- Maybe stock market investors

These criteria help identify potential patients who may benefit from implants and can afford to say yes to the treatment you recommend.

Once you have your list and have identified who you wish to do business with, it's time to craft your message. It doesn't matter where you focus your marketing efforts...whether you optimize your website, create a series of email sequences, or send a masterly crafted sales letter directly to your prospect's front door, the same rules apply. Your message must first grab and second hold their attention and, most importantly, have them ready to say yes before they scroll to the end or read the last word.

The biggest problem with selling a big-ticket service like dental implants is your best prospects are also your competitors best prospects. This means the second these high-value patients search for dental implants, visit a website, or show any form of traceable interest in what you sell, they are bombarded with pop-up ads, hunted by retargeting ads, and flooded with offers for free consultations.

The people who can benefit from the dental implants you offer the most, out of pure defense, have put up a wall to keep you away and turned a blind eye to the relentless assault of banner ads, pop-ups, and special offers thrust in front of them day after day.

As a consumer, you've undoubtedly experienced this. You show interest in purchasing something, maybe a new car, a vacation, or an air fryer, only to have your social media and news feeds carpet bombed with 0% financing offers and deals on airfare.

What do you end up doing? You tune this buzzing nonsense out and hit delete as fast as you can.

Your prospective patients are the same as you.

What does this mean for your business?

If you don't present yourself in a different light than all the rest, you never have a chance to connect on a personal level with the exact people who could give you a massive uptick in business, practically overnight.

Your marketing message must establish a relationship and build trust to connect with your ideal prospects. High-value prospects often like personal attention and hate the idea of "being sold" anything.

Master copywriter and direct marketing expert Russell Martino expounds on this. He says if you want to connect with high-value prospects who gladly buy and appreciate what you do for them, you must enter the conversation in their head. They need to know that you, not the three other dental practices in your community, are the trusted source for dental implants and their best choice to achieve the smile they've been dreaming of and the results they want most.

> ***"The goal of effective marketing is to make it easy for your customer to say yes."***
>
> ***- Russell Martino***

Getting past the barriers of B.S. is a problem. It's a big one. And until you solve it, you'll never build the kind of practice you imagined when you started.

Connecting with high-value clients is one of the highest ROI-generating and most effective ways to grow your practice.

So how do you do it? How do you break through the barriers and connect with high-value clients in a meaningful way?

I have an answer for you.

Over the past decades, I've surrounded myself with elite marketers and copywriters. These masters of persuasion guide my current marketing strategies and those of my clients. I, along with Dan Kennedy and Russell Martino, have developed a unique system to reach your best high-value prospects at the top of your prospect pyramid with nearly 100% accuracy. This system will get their attention and, most importantly, get them to respond.

This high-value patient marketing machine is simple and powerful. If you choose to work with eLaunchers, the entire process is done for you, but the rest of this chapter lays out the details of how you can achieve growth results on your own by crafting the right message and delivering it in a way that stands out.

This is a marketing tool that, with laser-guided accuracy, cuts through the clutter and, with full impact, empowers you to connect with your best high-value prospects.

> **It's more profitable to aggressively pursue a smaller number of high-value prospects than to go after a much larger number of average prospects.**

Identify high-value prospects and aggressively reach out to them with a tailor-made marketing message. You do this by developing a focused marketing effort to reach those prospects and transform them into satisfied patients eager to refer their friends and family to you for the dental implant-assisted smile of their dreams.

If you consistently attract high-value prospects, convert them into patients, and have them eagerly referring business to you, you have a patient marketing machine.

Still, how do you connect?

How Do You Break Through the B.S. Barrier?

If you show up looking like everyone else, expect to be ignored.

The average lost-in-the-inbox 21% email delivery rate and the microscopic 3% click-through rate is a recipe for failure—marketing suicide. Under the right circumstances, emails can be an effective marketing tool, but for the most part, unsolicited ads and emails are destined for the iconic trash can.

On the other hand, when you combine effective digital campaigns with powerful direct mail marketing, everything changes. Your High-Value Marketing Machine must include powerful marketing assets, including a master sales letter, a series of follow-up letters, web copy, and other copy assets designed to get your best high-value prospects to contact you essentially ready to buy.

But nothing happens until you grab their attention.

Let me ask you a question.

Do you know the open rate for a FedEx envelope? It's nearly 100%, and the direct mail delivery rates are almost as good.

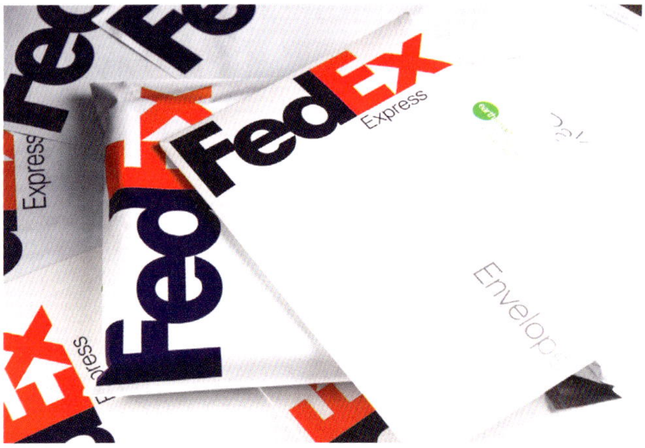

Now, put yourself in your ideal prospects' head. You hear a knock at your door, open and find a delivery driver in front of you, parcel in hand. You thank the man, take your parcel, and what? Do you instantly head to the nearest dustbin and toss it in? No. If you're like me, you're tearing into it the moment you shut your front door.

You've just effectively broken through the B.S. barrier.

Congratulations.

With some strategy and willingness to present yourself in a different light than everyone else, you can grab your ideal prospects' attention...that's the easy part.

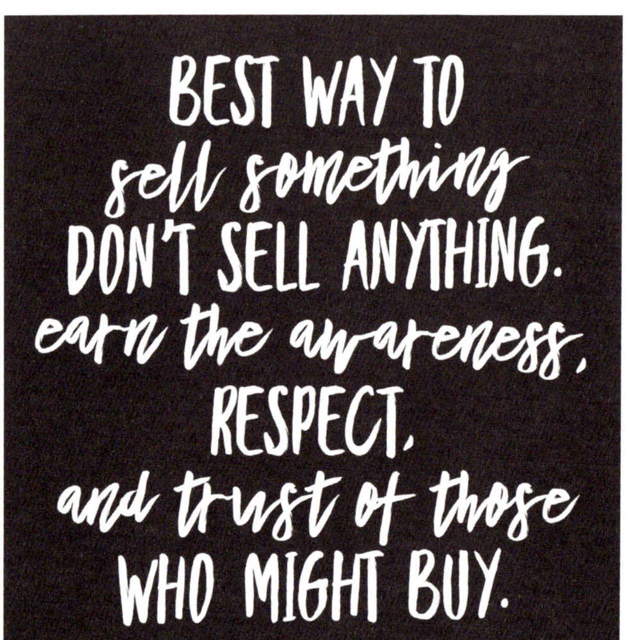

Now comes the real fun: Your message needs to do more than catch their attention. You want them to read every word and reach out to you with questions answered, objections handled, and essentially ready to do business.

CRAFT A MESSAGE THAT SELLS

Now it's time to sell.

And I don't mean to throw a bold SALE icon in front of them offering 10% off.

You want your message to feel like a conversation with a friend. This is not a hard sell. Your goal is persuasion, not a ramrod sales pitch.

You want your prospects to KNOW, LIKE and TRUST you.

If you want to sell anything, especially a high-value item like dental implants, you have to get into your prospects' head—address what they fear, whisper to their desires, and have them nodding yes from the moment they read the headline. You want them so engaged and intrigued that by the time they finish reading, they've already pulled out their phone to call for your next available appointment.

> *"If you want to create copy that sells, you have to grab your prospect's attention, hold it, and convince them that you have what they need."*
>
> \- Russell Martino

Tease a reward or hint at a danger.

Something like "The High Cost of Dental Neglect - Why Waiting Can Put Your Health and Finances at Risk."

Or maybe... "Your Smile, Your Confidence: The Connection You Can't Ignore."

When selling digitally or in print, it all starts with your headline. The headline must intrigue them. Otherwise, they won't read another word. You want a headline that invokes curiosity and captures their attention.

Once you pique their curiosity, it's time to deliver your masterly crafted message. An effective way to do this is by telling stories. Talk about a patient's transformation. Tell

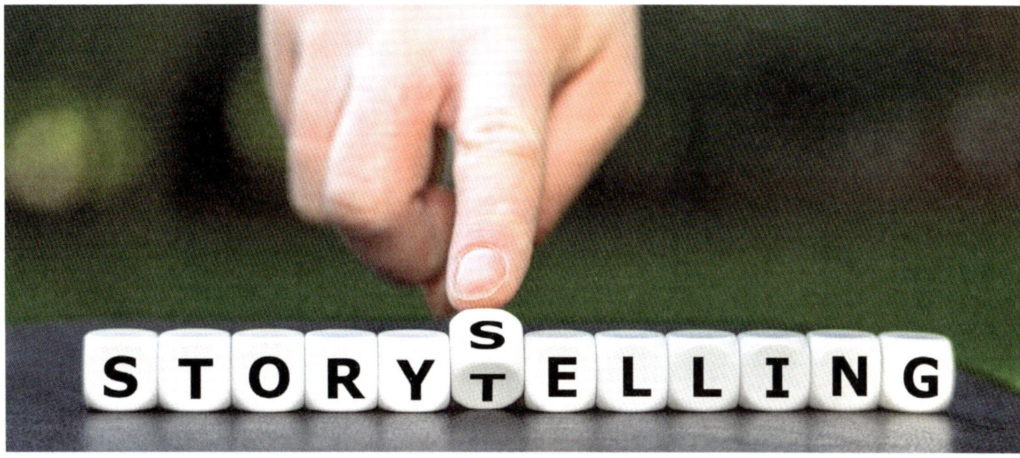

how they came to your office with a mouth full of missing or decayed teeth and walked out with the smile of their dreams. Talk about how this impacted their self-confidence, attractiveness and self-esteem. Tell your prospects about satisfied implant patients who may have similar stories to their own and with whom they can identify.

A good story helps hook them with emotion; providing valuable and informative content is what reels them in. Educate your patients on the benefits of choosing dental implants over dentures or other procedures. Explain the power of osseointegration and how dental implants fuse with the jawbone and promote bone regeneration, preserving the jawbone's integrity. Tell them if they choose dentures or do nothing to fix missing teeth, their jawbone will deteriorate, shrink and recede. Clearly explain why saying yes to dental treatment is the most effective way to optimize their oral health and have a radiant, confident smile they are proud of.

EDUCATE THEM

Give them all the reasons dental implants are the right choice for them.

TALK ABOUT:

- The regenerative nature of dental implants.
- How they feel and look like natural teeth.
- Research studies that show how a confident smile can improve their life.
- How safe and effective implants can permanently address missing, damaged or decayed teeth.
- The risk they take with their jawline if you choose dentures or do nothing to replace missing teeth.
- Cite research studies, mention peer-reviewed articles and provide evidence to back your claim. Don't overwhelm them with technical jargon; do dazzle them with details that establish your authority and credibility.

ADDRESS THEIR FEARS

Are they worried about looking unattractive or old before their time? Tell them by choosing dental implants, they never have to worry about looking like an old crone with a withered, shrunken face again.

Are they concerned about being judged for their disfigured teeth? Tell them the first-hand accounts, testimonies, and stories you've heard from happy dental implant patients who now have the world smiling back at them.

SPEAK TO THEIR DESIRES

Would they like to look 10 years younger, gain the attention of the opposite sex, or feel more confident when they speak, smile and laugh? Explain how an attractive, youthful smile is within reach if they choose dental implants.

ELIMINATE ALL DOUBT

Talk about lesser alternatives such as dentures and identify why they'll never work, as well as the benefits of dental implants. Talk about the risk they take by doing nothing and how easily and effectively they can fix the problems with their teeth and mouth with dental implants. Make it clear choosing your practice for their dental implants is the best move they can make because you and your team have the state-of-the-art techniques, tools and technologies to give them a radiant, confident smile that will last a lifetime. And back it all up with a guarantee.

CONFIRM THEIR SUSPICIONS

Dental implants are not cheap, and for good reason. They are custom-made for a patient's mouth. They are designed to last a lifetime, and they work to restore the jawline and promote oral health. They are an effective CURE for missing teeth. Besides, do patients want a cheaper, lesser alternative when it comes to their health?

You want to make an impression. You want your prospects to pay attention. You want them to know who you are and why your offer is valuable to them.

By delivering a persuasive message in the form of a sales letter and a series of follow-up letters, you will have top-of-the-mind awareness with your best prospects. You will have a rent-free room in their heads. They will feel like they know, like and trust you, even if you've never met.

And we all want to do business with people we like and trust.

A sales letter that sounds LESS like a sales letter and MORE like a conversation with a friend builds rapport and makes prospects feel like you know each other, even though you've never met.

You want your prospective implant patients to experience this when they read your letter. You want them to feel like they're having a conversation with a friend.

Effortlessly establish yourself as a trusted authority. Offer valuable insider insight into how you, the dental implant expert, can get results others can't because of training, state-of-the-art equipment, and the most up-to-date treatment and techniques. Give them a peek behind the curtains of your practice and introduce them to what sets you and your office uniquely above other dental practices.

So there it is—the secret ingredients to a persuasive sales message you can craft and duplicate time and again.

LET'S REVIEW:

- Deliver your sales message in a way that grabs their attention.
- Craft an engaging headline that piques their curiosity and captures their attention.
- Start with a story that pulls them in.
- Offer valuable content. Tell them what they have to gain and what they stand to lose.
- Address their fears.
- Tease their desires.
- Eliminate their doubt.
- Establish rapport and build authority and trust.
- Let them know why your practice is their best choice for dental implants.

There it is in a nutshell. There are countless books on persuasion from marketing legends, including Dan Kennedy and Russell Martino. I recommend ***The Ultimate Sales Letter*** by **Dan Kennedy** and ***What Makes Persuasive Sales Copy Persuasive*** by **Russell Martino**.

Remember, there is magic in your message. Effective direct mail marketing campaigns generate 3X and 10X increases in new dental implant income.

If you follow the formula outlined in this chapter, you'll likely land a slam dunk with your first mailing. If, on the other hand, the campaign falls short, you may need to spend more time with your message.

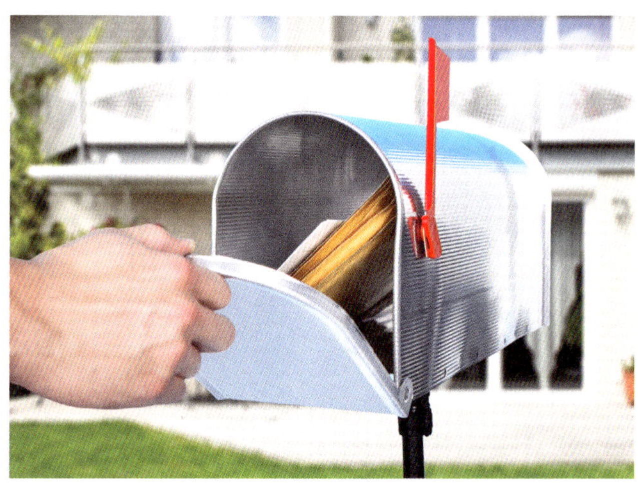

Now, if you're thinking to yourself, I'm a dentist, not a writer, and I don't know how to do ANY of that, you're in luck. Head to the resource section of this book. As I mentioned, I have examples of sales letters, compelling website copy and email campaigns with killer headlines and content you can use as a template. These examples give you the meat and potatoes; you just add the seasoning that resonates with you.

A master sales letter and series of shorter follow-up letters delivered to the homes of your ideal prospects is an effective way to throttle up sales that you can duplicate again and again. Use this message-to-market technique to connect with the diamonds in your database or a methodically selected list of your ideal prospects. Do this again and again any time you wish to see an uptick in your dental implant business.

Once you've hooked your prospects, capture their email and contact information as quickly as possible. Now, you can continue to communicate with them. If your print message persuaded them, they came to you presold and ready to say yes. Having their email address will let you communicate with them, keep them happy, and ask them for referrals.

If your prospect comes to you interested but not yet ready to say yes, then having an effective nurture campaign can turn tire kickers into buyers. We'll cover the power of a comprehensive growth strategy more in-depth in the following chapters, but for now, let your takeaway be this: The key to successfully managing all the components of your Marketing Machine is to keep your message consistent throughout—and your message needs to be all about your prospects. Your goal is to show them why they should sprint past your competitors and line up cash in hand, eager to achieve the smile of their dreams with the dental implants you provide.

Workbook

Message to Market Matters Workbook

To create a successful marketing campaign, you must connect the right message to the right market. In the last two chapters, we discussed how to identify your ideal prospects. By now, you should already have a list of ideal prospects you'd like to reach out to. Now, it's time to craft a message that resonates with them and has them eager to do business with you.

> *"The goal of effective marketing is to make it easy for your customer to say yes."*
>
> *- Russell Martino*

How to craft compelling copy that sells:

1. Grab their attention with a compelling headline.
2. Establish a relationship with your prospects, build trust and connect with them. You want them to know, like and trust you.
3. Your sales message should feel like a conversation with a friend, not a hard sell. The goal is persuasion, not a ramrod sales pitch.
4. Get into your prospects' head—address what they fear, whisper to their desires, and have them nodding yes from the moment they read the headline.
5. Identify problems they may not understand. Then, offer valuable insight and information that will enlighten them.

Use the worksheet below to help craft your message.

Headlines

In a world where attention is currency, headlines are your golden ticket to success. Headlines are not just a few bold words at the top of your letter. Your headline is the heartbeat of your content, the magnet for attention, and the catalyst for action. Master the art of a good headline, and watch as your message breaks through the clutter, leaving a lasting impression on your audience.

Some examples specifically for dental implants:

"Your Natural Beauty Restored with the Magic of Dental Implants"

Or "Invest in Your Smile: The Long-Term Value of Dental Implants"

Maybe "Rediscover Confidence - Transform Your Smile with Dental Implants!"

What dental treatment are you trying to sell with your copy? Who is the intended audience? What is on their minds and in their hearts? These things matter when crafting a great headline.

Establish trust and rapport with your patients.

Why should your patients trust you and see you as the authority in dentistry? Consider your degrees, education, accolades and awards. Have you written books? Been featured as a key-note speaker? Do you have glowing testimonials and case studies from satisfied patients?

Now let's dive deeper. What's your story? What got you into dentistry in the first place? Which patients are your favorite success stories? Why?

There is magic in STORYselling. So, be sure to have a few good ones. What stories can you tell your prospects to help them identify with you and trust you?

Think about your ideal prospects. What do they fear? Desire? Want? Need?

Are they afraid of looking old before their time because of missing teeth? Do they worry they'll be judged by ugly, disfigured teeth and shy away from social situations? Do they want to be seen as more attractive? Younger? More confident? What problems would you like to solve for your patients by helping them improve their smiles and the quality of their teeth?

Educate your patients and prospects.

What problems might your patients be suffering from without their knowledge? How can you shed light on their current situation and help them resolve problems they didn't know they had?

Here's an example: If your patients are missing teeth or suffering from gum disease, you know they are putting more than their oral health at risk. But they do not. This is where you come in. Educate them. Tell them what's really at stake when they decline recommended treatment.

Workbook

Give them additional reasons the dental treatment you recommend is right for them.

Here's an example. If you're talking about dental implants, discuss their regenerative nature, how they look and feel natural in the mouth, and so on. Talk about how, without a permanent solution to their missing teeth, patients can expect bone degeneration in their jaw and a cascade of negative health problems.

Whatever high-value treatments you recommend, be ready with a list of benefits they can expect by saying yes to that treatment and a list of consequences they may expect if they say no.

Once you've crafted a compelling message, use it to gain your prospects' attention. If you show up in an overstuffed inbox or a circular they're likely to throw away, your message will be lost. However, if your message shows up in a FedEx envelope, chances are high your prospect will pay attention. Yes, there is an extra cost for this, but if it means you attract more patients eager to say yes to high-end dentistry, it's worth it. If you've spent time with this workbook, you have the elements of a great sales message. If you still have concerns about creating this message yourself, go to my chapter on Samples and Swipe Files. I have examples of sales letters you can use to get your creative juices flowing.

With what you gathered in this chapter and the work you put into the workbook, you're ready to move on to the next step: Your Multimedia Message.

Chapter 5
Your Multimedia Message

Now it's time to create a personalized plan for measurable and consistent increases in profit. I'll cover:

a. Your multi-media message – reach your auditory, visual, and kinesthetic prospects.
b. How print and digital assets, in combination, can supercharge your ability to educate and entice potential patients.

In the last chapter, we discussed the importance of the message you deliver to your market. We discussed the importance of clearly identifying your ideal patients and crafting a marketing message that speaks to them. We talked about the importance of setting yourself apart and strategies to help you do that.

We dove into crafting a message that sells and the importance of enticing and educating prospective patients. How a persuasively crafted sales message must address your prospects' fears, speak to their desires, eliminate their doubts, and confirm their suspicions. You may have already homed in your message. Hopefully, the samples I provided in resources gave you a few ideas. You've likely got something good if you followed the formula I laid out in the last chapter.

This chapter and the two that follow are all about getting your dynamically crafted message to your audience through print and digital assets and ensuring your message resonates with your ideal patients and makes them eager to start treatment. The goal is to gain a sustainable competitive advantage for your practice.

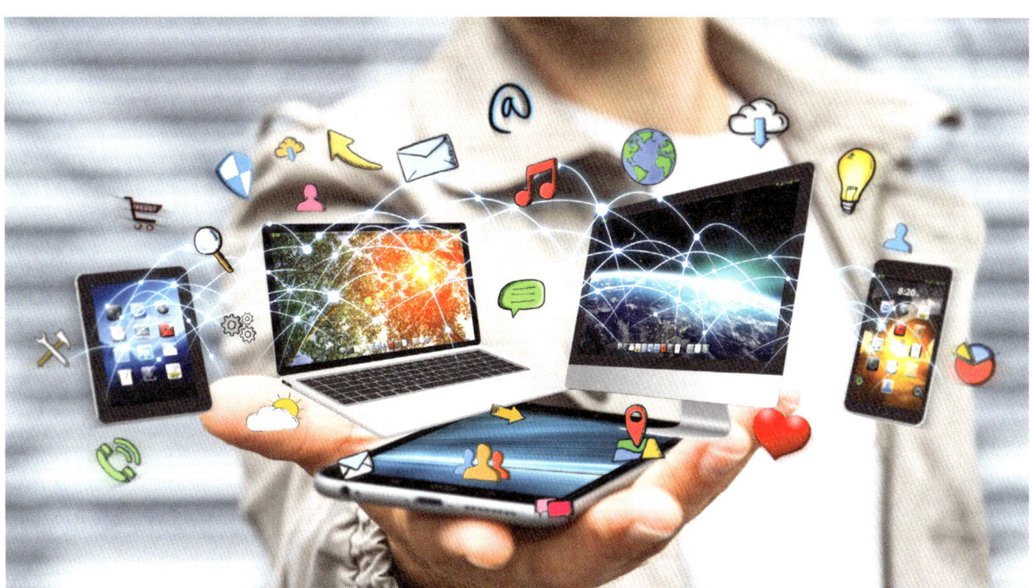

BUILD A MULTIMEDIA MESSAGE

When you build your marketing mix or your media package, be mindful of how different people will consume your information and prepare for all of it. Some only want to read. Some want to listen. Because different people respond to different media, you want a multimedia marketing campaign. Some of your prospects will be auditory learners, others visual and others kinesthetic. So, you want your message in audio, video, print, and an interactive format they can play with.

This may sound challenging, but it's much easier than you think.

The best way to build a multimedia message is to start with video. There are tablet video training programs that can teach you how to make a five- or six-minute video using your iPad. Just speak your message in front of your video recorder on your iPad and quickly edit your message using your iMovie app. Now you have your message on video.

Now, transcribe your video. You can do this yourself, or better yet, send it to a transcription company. Now, your message is on video and in print.

Take the video and convert it into an audio file, and now you have an audio message.

You can give the message transcript to an editor and graphic designer who can help you display it correctly. The audio file can go to your website or be placed on a CD you can give prospects with your letter. The message can go on a video book, your website or a DVD you can pass out.

How do you reach out to these premium patients? Most business owners think they must use radio, TV, mailers, SEO or social media ads. Some products and services sell like hotcakes in media like TV or radio. In fact, TV is a great way to sell hotcakes. IHOP TV ads show hot off-the-griddle pancakes with melted butter and maple syrup drizzled on top, bringing in breakfast lovers in droves.

Dental implants are not hotcakes.

NO ONE sees a 30-second commercial showing off attractive smiling people in a dentist's office and says, *"That's it; I didn't know anything about implants before, but now I know I'm ready to shell out $25,000 and have elective surgery. Count me in!"*

This just doesn't happen.

Plus, what percentage of a TV audience watching a sitcom on a Tuesday night will both need and be able to afford dental implants? Not many. MOST of your advertising budget would be lost on an audience with zero interest, need or ability to afford the implants you advertise. Radio ads may be worse than TV because you can't even show your audience those transformed smiles. SEO has its place, and mailers and social media ads can at least more effectively target an audience but still miss the mark when left on their own.

You can easily control your budget by keeping your message focused on your target audience. Instead of Facebook advertising or throwing out a commercial to the masses and casting a wide net, identify your narrowly selected market segment you want to go after and put together a multimedia, multitouch, micro-marketing campaign. Then, attack so fiercely your prospects either love or hate you but cannot ignore you. Go at it with everything you have. With a targeted, laser-focused micro-marketing campaign, you can concentrate your budget on bringing in only a fraction of the available market. The top 5% of your pyramid—the patients you want to do business with the most.

The trick is in the combination. When combined with effective landing pages, direct mail can be extremely powerful, and the cost to ROI can be easier to track and monitor.

The magic is in clarity. You need to be clear on what actions you want your prospects to take, and you need to guide them to the conclusion that contacting your office to schedule treatment is their next logical step.

Remember, not everyone will respond in the same way or at the same time. That's why it's important to have multiple channels of response.

Landing pages and sales funnels can be extremely effective channels of persuasion. Sales funnels and landing pages are like a magic journey that inevitably leads prospects to your dental chair. The journey starts when they hear about your dental practice and the great work you do with implants, either through a direct mail piece you send out, a targeted ad on social media, an email campaign, or word of mouth. They find the doorway (your landing page), a lot of great information about dental implants, and an irresistible offer for complimentary value-added content. This may be a special report, guide or e-book.

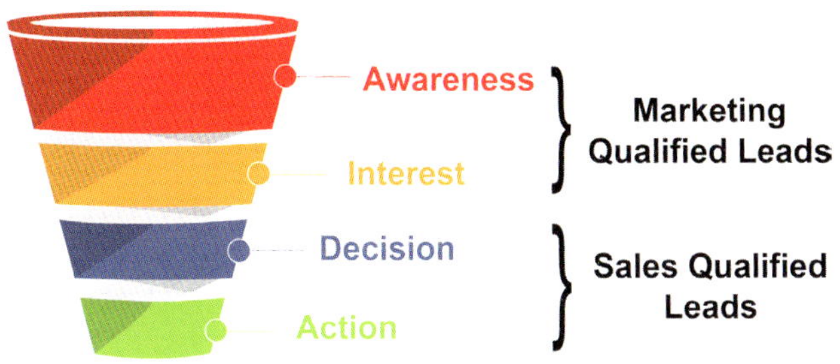

When they click on your offer, they get instant access to your valuable content. In Chapters 8 and 9, I'll walk you through what makes funnels wildly successful. In the resource tab, you can view my five most successful landing page campaigns, which generated more than $9 million in revenue for my clients. With this book, you have complete access to these pages. I recommend you study, imitate and emulate them to your heart's content. They are yours—my gift to you.

When your marketing efforts start to pay off and prospects contact you, don't ignore them. Have your persuasion theater ready. Track and measure what drives traffic to your landing page so you can turn up the heat on what's working and turn off what's not.

Have communication materials ready so you send information to prospects as soon as they request it. Be ready when they are. An automated landing page makes this seamless and effortless.

You need good bait if you want to catch the best fish. If you want your landing page to attract your ideal patients, you must entice them with something they want, need or will benefit from. So, what's your irresistible offer that will result in prospects trusting you and saying yes? What bait will you use in your masterly crafted sales message to entice them to take the next step? Maybe it's a book, a free report, a series of videos, or a piece of information about how dentistry can change their life. Perhaps it's a secret, something you know they probably aren't aware of but should be. You want an offer to please your prospects with no strings attached. If you are genuine and your message and offer meaningful, you will be a welcome guest, someone seen as an excellent human being volunteering their expertise and assistance.

Your marketing message, at this point, is just making prospects aware you have valuable information that WILL help them. The information is theirs for the taking, and all they need to do is share their name, email address, and phone number, and it will be given freely because you're just that great a person. The secret is you are, and the information you provide them is that great. The value-added content is real, and when your prospective patients finish absorbing it, they will know more and have more certainty about how dental implants can benefit them. Now, you are the trusted source with their best interest at heart.

THE TWO-STEP SQUEEZE

Your landing page is where you promote your value-added content and capture names, email addresses and phone numbers. As soon as prospects give you this information, take them to a secondary squeeze where you can say, *"Thank you for your request; here is the gift I promised. Now, if you give me your name and address, I have a special box or package to ship to you."* Some will say yes, and some won't, but you have another way of connecting with prospects who have a more kinesthetic learning style and would appreciate a tangible report instead of a digital download.

Plus, prospects who follow through on both calls to action represent more qualified leads. They were willing to share more information and told you what they needed. They are engaged with you and giving you a clear signal they are waiting for your advice.

Your prospects make their request, and you follow up with an email with a download link to your special report, guide, or other valuable content delivered to their inbox.

Some may request something tangible, so be ready with a promotional mailing. Maybe you send a handwritten letter, a video book, or a well-written sales letter accompanied by a three-dimensional knickknack. By doing this, you catch their attention. You show up differently than everyone else, making them more open to hearing about your offer.

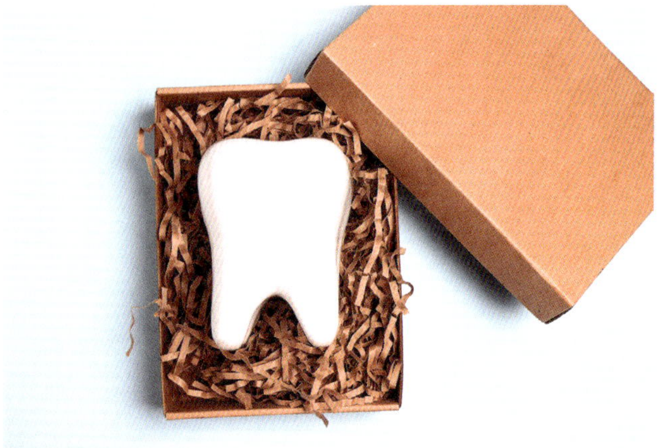

You should have respondent communications material ready for prospects requesting information you said would be readily available. Be ready when they are ready. You don't want to disappoint someone you are trying to build a relationship of trust with.

A consistent message is the key to success with a campaign like this. Once your marketing message and media are figured out, and you have carefully crafted and executed your approach, your target prospects will either ignore you or respond to you. If they ignore you, hit them again and again and again and again. People are busy. They might have overlooked the first attempt, so don't give up. If you've researched who you want to go after, you know your target market is good. You've got to spend more time, energy and resources to provide enough touchpoints. It takes up to seven or eight touches to get someone's attention. If it takes more than one or more than three or seven attempts to get their attention, keep at it. Chase them until they see you and respond.

When prospects raise their hand and say yes, please acknowledge them and give them the gift you promised. Follow through on your promises and take action when you should. If your offer is engaging and the content you give them valuable, you will shift their minds in your direction. If you continue to engage them, the chances of them agreeing to treatment increase.

Instead of giving away your physical book, report, CD, or DVD for free, you can create a **self-liquidating offer (SLO).** You will send them a book, a DVD or a whole bunch of information about the technology behind dental implants, and all they have to do is cover the cost of postage. This is a nice offer, and many people will respond to it.

What you're doing is clearly identifying an interested buyer. It's one thing to say, "Sure, yeah, send me your stuff." But if they pull out a credit card and spend a few dollars to receive your package, this signals they're the real deal. The idea is to get an initial respondent to agree to a small transaction or micro-commitment.

Dr. Charlie Martin calls this concept "Experience the Genius."

THE TRIAD: KNOW, LIKE AND TRUST

We covered much of this in the previous chapter, but it bears repeating.

Once a prospect has agreed to accept your offer, received your digital download, or received your promotional package, it's time to establish the triad—know, like and trust (KLT). People buy from people they like, and people will like you if they can trust you. So, when your ideal prospects are absorbing your special report, e-book, or value-added content, make sure you hit on the big three. When they finish, you want them to know you, like you and trust you.

Everyone's definition of trust is different. You must establish trust in a way they find meaningful.

What can you do to establish trust? First, ask yourself, what kind of information do your prospective patients crave? What web pages do they visit? What ads do they respond to? What questions did they ask on an initial call? What source referred them to you? Or, if you have them on the phone, ask them point-blank if they want to know more about the science and technology behind dental implants, or how dental technologies have advanced and changed over the last decade. Maybe they'd like to learn more about periodontal disease, or have another area of concern. With a little effort, you could have an eight-to-10-page special report tailored to each potential concern ready to give out, for free, upon request.

You want prospects to get to know you and to like you, so speak to them as you would a friend or confidant. Tell them why you're passionate about dentistry. Talk about your aha moment when you discovered the life-changing effects of dental implants. Discuss your favorite patient stories and the transformations and renewed self-confidence you've witnessed after restoring their vibrant smiles.

You want to share information that speaks directly to their challenges while simultaneously establishing trust in the relationship. An effective way to do this is with testimonials from happy, satisfied dental implant patients. Somewhere in your report, include Google reviews or reference a book you wrote. (You might be amazed at how easy it is to become a "best-selling author" on Amazon.)

So now, you've delivered your message along with your value-added content. You've proven to your prospects you are a trusted authority with their best interest in mind. You've addressed their fears, confirmed their suspicions, eliminated their doubts, and shown them a better way. Now that you've done all this, is it time to ask for the sale?

You don't want to be quick to ask for an order. If you try to monetize a relationship before the trust level has solidified, it will backfire. In today's world, people want information now and in the way they want it. That is what consumers expect. Our digitally connected lives have us eager for instant gratification. You have to understand how your prospective patients capture, analyze, understand, read and respond to information. Trust is not magic or voodoo. If you know who you are, who you are for, how you want to help your patients and understand if they want to be helped in that way, you will have them taking the next step.

It's OK to extend an offer for prospects to contact you, but you don't need to make this a hard sale. If you've crafted your message and valuable content correctly, your prospective patients will know you, like you, trust you, and, most importantly, see you as the only one who can expertly give them the results they want with the transformative magic of dental implants.

I hope you can see the power of combining digital and print assets. I assure you, though, this is just a taste of what's to come. In the following chapters, we will dive deep and explore the specifics of how to craft a variety of print and digital assets that establish you as the authority on dental implants and the only one your prospects will ever consider trusting to makeover or restore their smiles.

Workbook

Your Multimedia Message Workbook

A simple way to build a multimedia message is to start with video. There are tablet video training programs that can teach you to make five- or six-minute videos using your iPad. Just say your message in front of your iPad's video recorder and quickly edit it using the iMovie app. Now, you have your message on video.

Then, transcribe your video. You can do this yourself, or better yet, send it to a transcription company. Your message will now be on video and in print.

Take the video and convert it into an audio file, and now you have an audio message.

Give your message's transcript to an editor and graphic designer who can help you display it correctly. The audio file can go to your website or be placed on a CD to give out with your letter. The message can go on a video book, your website, or a DVD you can pass out.

Use this section to brainstorm. What message do you wish to convey to your potential patients?

Would you like them to know the benefits of dental implants? The risks they take if they do not properly treat gum disease? Review what we discussed in the previous chapter and craft a message that resonates with your potential patients. With a little effort, this message can be easily turned into the script you use to craft your multimedia message.

LANDING PAGES AND SALES FUNNELS

These web pages are set up to take your prospect on a journey. At the beginning, they're directed to a landing page or sales funnel through targeted social media ads, postcards, or maybe a direct mail campaign. A landing page might be designed to capture prospect names, emails, phone numbers and addresses by getting them to download a free report or e-book.

You can instantly supply a free report, e-book or podcast with a downloadable link. Prospects may request a tangible product, so have one ready. This is an excellent opportunity to capture their physical address and WOW them.

Create a package for your prospects that shows them you are not just an average dentist. You care. You go above and beyond. You are the one they should trust with their dental needs. Your package should include a main product like a special report, book or CD of your podcast, a sales letter, a special offer such as a gift certificate, and maybe a small gift. I go over this type of package in detail in later chapters when I discuss shock and awe packages. Check out my chapter on Samples and Swipe Files for more information on how to put this together.

For now, do a bit of brainstorming on what might go into a package you send to a prospective patient.

A sales funnel might be designed to get them to sign up for a free consultation.
If you wish to create a landing page, what is your offer? Do you have a free report? An e-book? Maybe recordings of your podcast or YouTube series? What is your irresistible, free offer that makes your prospects eager to learn more?

If you wish to create a sales funnel, consider your offer. If prospects agree to a free dental implant consultation, for example, you could offer them a $250 gift certificate they can use toward a recommended treatment plan. Think about what incentive you can offer to make your prospects eager to say yes.

Combining digital and print assets has great power. You've glimpsed a taste of it so far, and there's more to come in the following chapters and workbooks.

Chapter 6
Selling in Print Part I

Your step-by-step guide to creating and implementing print assets that pre-sell your ideal patients on doing business with you.

In a world where consumers are bombarded with information and misinformation every time they open their email or search the web, print assets give you a way to stand out from the crowd of competition.

Your first point of contact through print may be the sales letter we discussed in previous chapters. A well-crafted persuasive sales letter delivered via FedEx to a well-researched list of prospects is a powerful marketing asset. But that is just the beginning. Print assets can be used throughout the patient acquisition process.

When properly constructed and delivered, print assets are powerful tools that help establish your authority, answer your prospects' questions, handle their objections, and entice them to say yes to the treatment you recommend.

> ***"I've learned that people will forget what you said, people will forget what you did, but people will never forget how you made them feel."***
>
> **- Maya Angelou**

THE POWER OF SHOCK AND AWE

Marketing guru Dan Kennedy says "shock and awe" boxes are an effective strategy for engaging with prospects and converting them into patients—getting them excited about you and ensuring you're standing out from your competition.

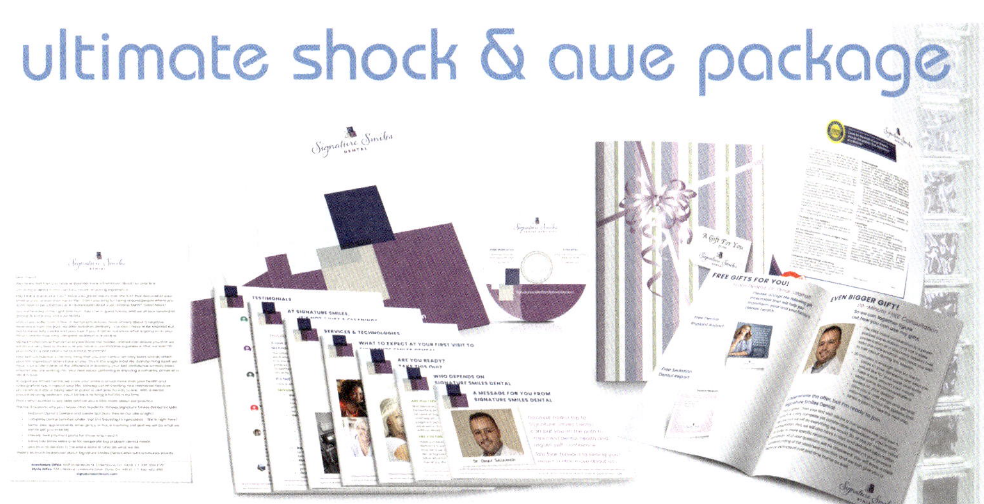

When prospects reach out to you and says they are interested in your services, a shock and awe package can be the next step in the journey that leads them to agreeing to and beginning treatment.

Dental implant patients are perfect candidates to receive, benefit from and respond to shock and awe packages. Here's why. For these patients to reap the benefits of dental implants, they must first agree to a substantial upfront cost and then undergo elective surgery.

If you asked just about anyone if they'd like to shell out a small fortune and agree to elective surgery, no one's going to raise their hand—that is, of course, unless they know the transformative effects of a brilliant smile are waiting for them on the other end.

This is where a shock and awe package comes in. These packages are an extremely effective method of turning lookers into buyers and ensuring those who agree to an appointment follow through.

The Shock and Awe Experience

Just imagine.

Prospective patients might reach out to you after reading your sales letter, seeing an online ad, or being referred by a friend. These prospects are in the beginning stage of interest in dental implants but not yet ready to commit.

A few days later, the doorbell rings and a UPS driver is at the doorstep with a Fed-Ex package in hand. Their interest is immediately piqued. Do they drop the box on the entryway table and go back to what they were doing? That's doubtful. Odds are they tear open the package the moment the front door clicks back into place.

Now you have their attention.

They open your package and are greeted by a personalized cover letter that mentions them by name, thanks them for their interest in your dental practice, and explains what's inside the package they just received. Maybe you include a nice journal with your practice's logo on it in case they wish to take notes, or a deluxe sugar-free cookie in the shape of a tooth they can enjoy while exploring the package. Include a copy of your book if you have one or create a special report on dental implants.

Adding tangible items increases your credibility and the perceived value of your package. It is also seen as both generous and fun.

Now comes the important part—the structural components that make up an informative and persuasive shock and awe package. After prospects read your cover letter and eat your cookie, it's time to get down to business. Ultimately, a shock and awe package is a sales presentation, but you don't want it to be perceived as one, at least not right away. This is a soft sales package aimed at informing your prospects, answering their questions, easing their fears, and removing their doubts. As they go through this package, you want them to effortlessly come to the conclusion that agreeing to dental implants at your practice is the best decision they can make.

Don't start with a hard sales pitch; instead, ease into the conversation going on in your prospect's head.

The Anatomy of a Shock and Awe Package

The Pocket Folder

The pocket folder houses your material and should match your established branding guidelines with your logos clearly visible. The pocket folder can be placed in a clear plastic envelope and placed right alongside the package's swag.

Statement of Guarantee

This is a single-page statement of guarantee/risk reversal. Here, you demonstrate how you eliminate almost all risks for your client. You show that you, too, have skin in the game and will not take their money and run.

The guarantee piece is something your existing clients will talk about to their friends they want to refer to you. You do not have to guarantee performance. All you have to guarantee is you will do what you say.

Everyone can offer SOME guarantee.

Gift Brochure

This is one of the most important elements of the shock and awe package. In this piece, you lead by discussing the tangible gifts you've included in your package, maybe your book or free report on the benefits of dental implants, or maybe it's a set of CDs talking about how implant technology has evolved over the years. The biggest gift you will give them is a free smile consultation, where they will receive a comprehensive exam and time to talk with you about dental implants and if they are a good candidate.

The Right Pocket

THERE ARE SEVEN ELEMENTS THAT GO IN THE RIGHT POCKET:

- A Message From...
- Who Depends On
- Are You Ready? Take the Quiz
- About Your Free Consultation
- Services and Technologies
- Meet the Team
- Testimonials and Case Studies

Each element is a stand-alone sales tool. These marketing assets clarify who you are, who you help and what you do. They provide social proof that your patients love their smiles and that they agreed to treatment with you. Here's a closer look at the seven elements:

1. A Message From...

This is your personality brochure.

Here, you talk about who you are, why you do what you do, why implant dentistry is important to you, who you want to serve, and how what you do is different than all the other dentists they can choose from. Here, you'll give your origin story, discuss your core strengths, and tell them how you became so good at implant dentistry. This is about more than just listing your credentials. Tell them about when you realized you wanted to be a dentist. Tell them about the joy you get from transforming smiles and giving people back the ability to smile and enjoy life on a level they've been missing for so long. Here, you want to establish yourself as a trusted, likable authority who has their best interests at heart.

2. Who Depends On

This is where you describe your ideal patient. You want your readers to find themselves in this description. You want to talk about how moms, dads and grandparents depend on you, how anyone who recently lost a tooth or has a mouth full of dental problems depends on you, how anyone who wishes to look 10 years younger and restore their ability to eat the foods they love depends on you.

Explain WHY you seek out these types of clients, how you serve them, what you do better than anyone, and why you are the trusted source of dental implants and the most qualified dentist to give them the smile they deserve.

3. Are you Ready? Take the Quiz

This interactive piece allows your prospect to self-qualify or disqualify themselves in their own mind so they come prepared to make a deal. "Pain" questions such as, *"Do you shy away from mirrors and avoid social situations because you are unhappy and embarrassed about your disfigured smile or missing teeth?"* create awareness and agitate the need. Follow up with questions like *"Are you ready to regain your youthful smile and confidence with straight white teeth that look and feel natural in your mouth and have your friends and family showering you with compliments?"*

By the time someone completes a well-structured leading quiz, they will have run a gambit that hits on all the emotional hot buttons, from the pain they'll experience if they decline treatment to the joy and rewards they'll reap if they agree right away. This quiz can be used as a stand-alone, self-qualifying sales presentation powerful enough to get any viable prospects' attention and bring them to the table IF they are, in fact, a good candidate for dental implants.

4. About Your Free Consultation

Here, rules of engagement for the initial consultation are defined. Talk about what prospects can expect from the moment they walk through your practice door to the time they will spend consulting with you at the dentist's chair. Discuss how their questions will be answered and their concerns addressed. By the time it's over, they will know with certainty if dental implants are right for them.

Always REVEAL a price range in writing. It is important they know what they are getting themselves into. Obviously, with dental implants, each patient will have unique needs. There is no one price-fits-all answer, but if they understand the ballpark amount they can expect, they won't be shocked later.

5. Services and Technologies

This is where you highlight and present your dental implant, cosmetic and periodontic services. You discuss the oral health problems you treat and how you do this better than anyone else. Maybe you mention your state-of-the-art facilities, high-resolution imaging, or 3D printing in-house lab. Maybe you discuss the extensive training you and your team have undergone to become the undisputed expert authority on dental implants. You can discuss everything from single-tooth implants to full-mouth restorations and cosmetic makeovers. If you specialize in mini-dental implants or specific methods of implant placement, this is where you go into detail and explain why this is important to them.

6. **Meet the Team**

You want your prospective patients to feel welcome and at home. When they come in for an initial consultation, you want them to see faces they recognize. You want them to know everyone in your practice is an expert who has their best interest in mind. Highlight what sets you and your team apart in the world of dentistry. You want you and your staff to be seen not just as a dental team, but as trusted friends.

7. **Testimonials and Case Studies**

This should be eight to 12 pages, depending on how many testimonials and case studies you have.

This can include pictures of happy patients, before and after images, and images of handwritten letters if you have handwritten testimonials. If you have great transformation stories, add them here.

This section is a celebratory document that offers social proof in the form of happy patients and smiling faces.

On the final page of this section, ask prospects to reach out to you to schedule their smile consultation.

"Be our next success story!"

Your shock and awe package is a way to exceed your prospects' expectations, engage their interests, and build their loyalty. The idea is to make going through the package seem like opening a present. Although they can range in price from costly to downright expensive, they are a great way to spend your marketing dollars. If you've done your due diligence with your list research, then you are offering this package to a select and qualified group of ideal prospective patients who have already shown interest in you. Shock and awe packages are extremely effective at cutting through clutter, demanding attention and being memorable.

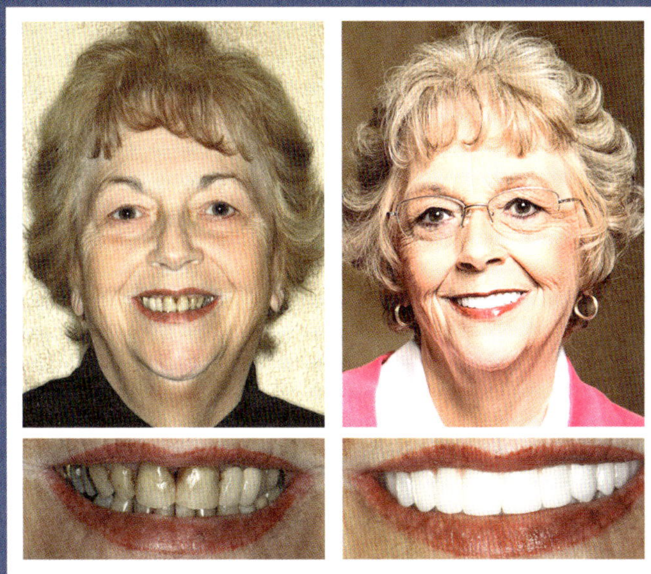

Judy

Judy had suffered, for many years, with recurrent decay and sensitive teeth. Nearly every tooth had decay, and she was tired of multiple fillings. The decay had moved down around her gum line and under her gums, and her teeth were essentially non-restorable. She chose the route of the implant-supported zirconia bridge. This is such a predictable, beautiful way to restore her mouth and, as Judy will tell you, these just feel like real teeth.

Bill

Bill had a history of breaking multiple teeth. He had moderate to severe tooth wear and a misalignment of his jaw joints and teeth. His powerful chewing muscles were locked up and over-stressed.

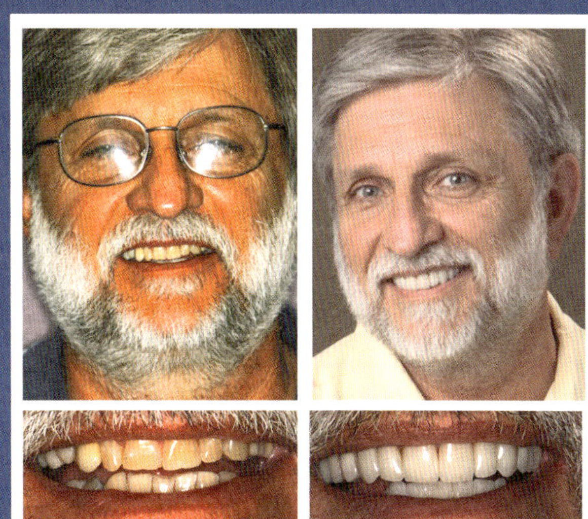

The stresses cause teeth, crowns and bridges to break repeatedly. Once his system was realigned and his teeth were built to naturally fit his jaw joints and how his muscles and body wanted to move, the pattern of breaking teeth ended.

This is another case where you can really see it in the eyes and the rest of his face. How much more relaxed he is once the right joint position and the right bite were found.

Selling in Print Part I Workbook

Your first point of contact through print may be the sales letter we discussed in Chapter 5. A well-crafted persuasive sales letter delivered via FedEx to a well-researched list of prospects is a powerful marketing asset. But that is just the beginning. Print assets can be used throughout the patient acquisition process.

THE POWER OF SHOCK AND AWE

What goes in your shock and awe package? Let's brainstorm some ideas here. Be sure to refer back to the Sample and Swipe File Chapter for examples.

The Pocket Folder

This should match your established branding guidelines with your logos clearly visible. The pocket folder can be housed in a clear plastic envelope right alongside the package's swag content.

Statement of Guarantee

A single-page statement of guarantee/risk reversal: Everyone can guarantee something. Clearly explain how you stand behind your products and treatment. What certainty can you offer prospective patients?

Gift Brochure

In this piece, discuss the tangible gifts you've included in your package. This could be your book or free report about the benefits of dental implants, or perhaps it's a set of CDs discussing how implant technology has evolved over the years. The biggest gift you will give prospects is a free smile consultation that includes a comprehensive exam and time with you to determine if they are a good candidate for dental implants.
What is your irresistible offer for prospective patients?

A Message From...

This is your personality brochure.
What's your story? What message do you wish to share with prospective patients?
This is about more than just listing your credentials. Tell them how you realized you wanted to be a dentist. Tell them about the joy you get from transforming smiles and giving people the ability to smile and enjoy life on a level they've been missing for so long. Here, you want to establish yourself as a trusted, likable authority who has your patients' best interests at heart.

Who Depends On

You want your readers to find themselves in this description. You want to talk about how moms, dads and grandparents depend on you, how anyone who recently lost a tooth or has a mouth full of dental problems depends on you, how anyone who wishes to look 10 years younger and restore their ability to eat the foods they love depends on you.

Explain WHY you seek out these types of clients, how you serve them, what you do better than anyone, and why you are the trusted source of dental implants and the most qualified dentist to give them the smile they deserve.

Are you Ready? Take the Quiz

This interactive piece allows prospects to self-qualify or disqualify themselves in their own mind so they come prepared to make a deal. "Pain" questions such as, *"Do you shy away from mirrors and avoid social situations because you are unhappy and embarrassed about your disfigured smile or missing teeth?"* are asked to create awareness and agitate the need. Follow up with questions like, *"Are you ready to regain your youthful smile and confidence with straight white teeth that look and feel natural in your mouth and have your friends and family showering you with compliments?"*

What questions do you want your patients to consider?

1.
2.
3.
4.
5.
6.
7.
8.
9.
10.

About Your Free Consultation

Talk about what patients can expect from the moment they walk through your practice door to the time they spend consulting with you. Discuss how their questions and concerns will be answered. By the time it's over, they will know with certainty if dental implants or the high-end dental treatment you recommend are right for them.

Be sure to mention the price here. This will save sticker shock reactions and aggravation later on.

Services and Technologies

Highlight and present your dental implant, cosmetic and periodontic services here. Discuss the oral health problems you treat and how you do this better than anyone else. Maybe mention your state-of-the-art facilities, high-resolution imaging or 3D printing in-house lab. Discuss the extensive training you and your team have undergone to become the undisputed expert authority on dental implants. You can discuss everything from single-tooth implants to full-mouth restorations and cosmetic makeovers. If you specialize in mini-dental implants or specific methods of implant placement, this is where you go into detail and explain why this is important to them.

What sets you apart? What makes your practice unique? What advantage do your patients receive by choosing you?

Meet The Team

From your hygienist to yourself, highlight what sets you and your team apart in dentistry. You want your staff to be seen as a dental team and as trusted friends. Paint this picture in the Meet the Team section.

Testimonials and Case Studies

This will have eight to 12 pages depending on the number of testimonials and case studies you have. Include pictures of happy customers, before and after images, and images of hand-written letters if you have them. If you have great transformation stories, add them here. Who are your favorite success stories?

Spend some time with this workbook, and you will have the elements you need to create a compelling shock and awe package.

Workbook

Chapter 7
Selling in Print Part II

In the first part of Selling in Print, we covered the power of shock and awe, a sales piece that stands alone and converts your prospects into patients. Your case presentation is like a shock and awe package, but one with the power to turn any team member into a master salesperson.

YOUR CASE PRESENTATION: A MASTER SALESMAN IN A BOX

This powerful asset is a conversion tool that allows any team member, from your hygienist to your receptionist, to deliver a powerful sales presentation.

While shock and awe packages are sent to prospects before the appointment, the case presentation package is handed to them on arrival and used as a conversation prop at their consultation.

Elements of a persuasive case presentation include:

Audio CD or Video DVD

This is an important element of a case presentation package.

Frequently asked questions should be answered in your audio CD or video DVD. and objections handled. Prospects will clearly understand what they need, what they get, and why you are the right choice for them.

You can write your script or hire an expert copywriter to develop a script for an audio CD or a video DVD. Arranging for someone to interview you is a great way to do this. During the interview, discuss your dental practice, implants, and why prospects should agree to treatment you recommend.

Patients walk out with the case presentation package, regardless if they agree to treatment. If they said yes, this CD/DVD serves as a tool to handle buyer remorse. If they

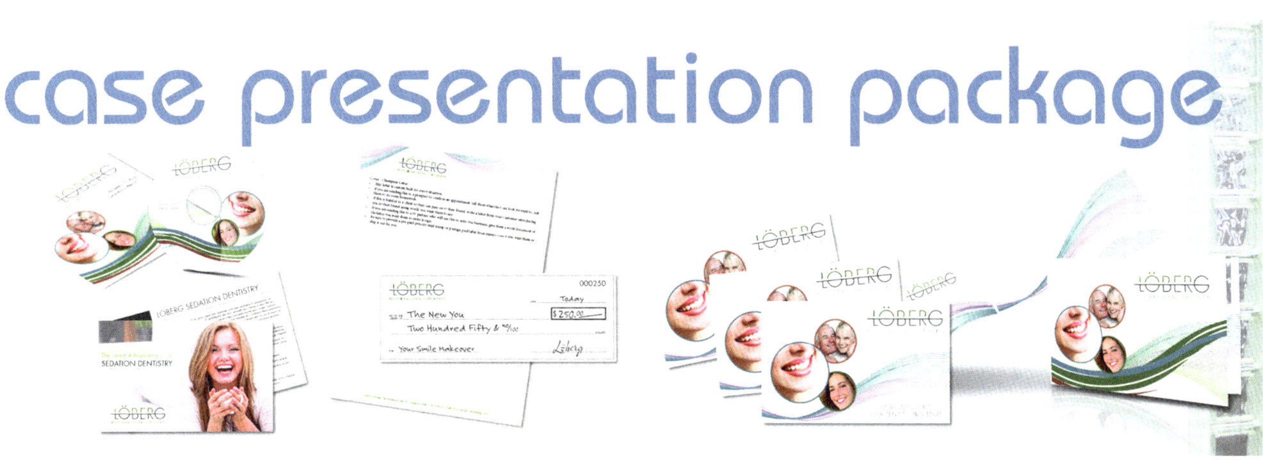

walk out saying, "I'll have to think about it," (appointment no sale), this audio or audio-visual element is designed to bring them back for a follow-up appointment where you can answer their questions.

Check or Gift Voucher

The gift voucher should have a substantial face value ($250, for example) that prospects can use toward the implant procedure or treatment plan you recommend. Offering the gift voucher tells them this will be a sizable purchase and today is the day they will be buying. They will recognize you're giving them a small token of appreciation for spending time with you. This is money in their pocket they can spend on YOU.

Letter to Customer

This is a champion letter from YOU to your patients, thanking them for their interest in dental implants or the treatment you recommend. It starts with "Congratulations, I am glad you took this step. Then, discuss the pain they will avoid and the benefits they will gain if they follow through.

Postcard

A postcard is an executive summary document describing the benefits of the proposed treatment or program. This visual represents their life AFTER they agree to an implant procedure or your recommended treatment.

Step-By-Step Guide

This step-by-step process flowchart details what patients can expect during their scheduled treatments. The purpose is to future-pace prospects and get them to see themselves starting their implant procedure, to set expectations, define rules of engagement, and have them thinking about the long-term results they will achieve once their oral health problems have been corrected and they're grinning from ear to ear with two rows of healthy looking, straight teeth.

Treatment/Service Options

This multi-page booklet describes (with pictures, illustrations and text) your patients' options. Options are important. If you don't give them enough options to pick from, they will seek a second opinion from someone else and see if YOU are the right option. You are helping them choose within a controlled environment by giving them options. This may include less expensive treatment options, such as dentures and bridges. Compare and contrast these options with implants and discuss how saving money on a lesser treatment could have long-term costs they will not want to pay later.

Testimonials

The testimonials section of your case presentation will be similar to what you have in your shock and awe package. This is where you offer social proof. Include pictures of happy patients with before and after images. Add your transformation stories here as well. Again, this celebratory document offers social proof through happy patients and smiling faces. On the final page of this section, ask them to say yes. *"Be our next success story!"*

With a compellingly crafted case presentation, anyone in your office can answer your patients' questions, ease their doubts, speak to their dreams and desires, and get them to say yes to treatment.

Power in Print: Additional Assets That Turn Prospects into Patients.

A masterly crafted sales letter paired with a shock and awe package and case presentation will put you miles ahead of your competition.

Additional print assets that can and do ring the cash register for practice owners include:

1. **Smile Books.** These bound books feature glossy pictures and dozens of before and after photos of happy patients who first showed up to your office with a mouth full of decayed or damaged teeth and left with two rows of brilliant, straight teeth that look and feel natural in their mouths. This book also can act as an educational piece that informs patients about what will happen to their jawbone if they do not replace missing teeth. You can discuss the impact dental implants will have on their oral and overall health, as well as their options for treatment—all with lovely glossy photos, of course.
2. **Automated Holiday Greeting Cards and Birthday Cards.** Everyone loves getting a card during the holidays or on their birthday, even if it's from the dentist. Greeting cards are a great way to stay in touch with your patients and can serve as a gentle reminder to attend their annual, semiannual or quarterly recommended treatment at your office.
3. **Dental Patient Experience Assets.** An easy way to turn satisfied patients into raving fans is by giving them a

little extra. This might come in the form of a new patient welcome box, an end-of-treatment celebration box, or a thank you for referral gift. These gifts do not need to be elaborate; they can be something small you can put together that shows you care. A welcome box might contain an oral hygiene kit, dental health literature, an appointment reminder magnet, or a notepad. A celebration box might contain a congratulatory box, sugar-free gourmet treats, and a glossy set of their before and after pictures.

4. **B-2-B Referral Boxes.** These go to general dentists, doctors or other professionals with patient lists similar to yours who can refer you patients. This package may look similar to a shock and awe package, but it is tailored more to the professional than the patient. In this box, include a copy of your book (if applicable), special reports, a personalized goody bag, and some brochures or literature they can offer their patients.
5. **Postcards and Greeting Cards**. These can be an effective, cost-efficient way to reach your patients and solicit new ones. While postcards typically do not perform as well as a well-crafted sales letter, they can be a great way to gain momentum in a sales funnel that asks prospects to scan a QR code or go to your website and download a free report. Remember, you cannot send postcards to your patients, as any communication from a doctor must be enclosed in a sealed envelope to protect patient privacy. For patient communications, use greeting cards that come in envelopes. Postcards should be used only for prospects.

The print assets you choose for your practice will likely give you an advantage over competitors who rely only on digital marketing assets. Sure, they can cost more to produce, but if your message is strong and your market is hot, the ROI is worth it every time.

I'm sure by now you can see how having a strong arsenal of print assets can make a difference in your practice.

You'll stand out in the eyes of your patients and your community, and gain more referrals because you will create an experience that people feel good about—and how you make people feel is what they remember most.

Selling in Print Part II Workbook

YOUR CASE PRESENTATION: TURN ANY TEAM MEMBER INTO A MASTER SALESPERSON

A solid case presentation can turn any team member into a master salesperson. What goes in your case presentation? Let's brainstorm some ideas. Be sure to refer back to the Sample and Swipe File Chapter for examples.

Audio CD or Video DVD

You want to address frequently asked questions in your audio CD or video DVD and for prospects to clearly understand what they need, what they get, and why you are the right choice for them.

Arranging for someone to interview you is a great way to put this together. During the interview, discuss your dental practice, implants, and other high-end dental procedures and why prospects should agree to your recommended treatment.

Spend a few minutes here brainstorming what you may want to say. Consider having multiple versions of this media, with one on dental implants, one on gum disease, one on cosmetic dentistry, etc.

Check or Gift Voucher

Include a special offer in the form of a gift voucher or check for a substantial amount, at least $250, that patients can use toward the treatment you recommend. Make sure the offer has an expiration date.

Letter to Customer

This is a champion letter from YOU to your patients, thanking them for their interest in the treatment you recommended. It starts with ”Congratulations, I am glad you took this step. Then, discuss the pain they will avoid and the benefits they will gain if they follow through. What do you wish to say to your prospective patients?

Postcard

A postcard is an executive summary document describing the benefits of the proposed treatment or program. This visual represents life AFTER patients agree to an implant procedure or your recommended treatment.
What ideas would you like to add to this postcard?

Step-By-Step Guide

This step-by-step process flowchart details what patients can expect during their scheduled treatments.

Treatment/Service Options

This multi-page booklet describes (with pictures, illustrations and text) your patients' options. This may include less expensive treatment. Compare and contrast these options.

Testimonials

The testimonials section of your case presentation will be similar to the one in your shock and awe package. This celebratory document offers social proof through happy patients and smiling faces.

Additional print assets that can and do ring the cash register for practice owners include:

1. **Smile Books.** These bound books feature glossy pictures and dozens of before and after photos. They also can act as an educational piece.

   Which patients would you like to showcase in your smile book?

   ____
   ____
   ____
   ____

2. **Dental Patient Experience Assets.** An easy way to turn satisfied patients into raving fans is by offering that little extra. This might come in the form of a new patient welcome box, an end-of-treatment celebration box, or a thank you for referral gift.

   What would you like to add to your patient experience package?

   ____
   ____
   ____
   ____

3. **B-2-B Referral Boxes.** These go to general dentists, doctors or other professionals with patient lists similar to yours and can refer you patients. This package may look like a shock and awe package, but it is tailored more to the professional than the patient.

   What elements would you add to your B-2-B referral box?

   ____
   ____
   ____
   ____

The print assets you choose for your practice will likely give you an advantage over competitors who rely only on digital marketing assets.

Workbook

Chapter 8
Your Digital Empire Part I: Make Your Online Assets Work for You

I find it funny, most of us have lived long enough to witness the birth of the internet. We remember the novelty of it and how exciting it was to check our inbox and find an email waiting. Back then, our physical mailboxes were littered with junk mail, but our emails were precious.

Alas, those days are gone. The novelty of the internet wore thin long ago. And "clearing out email" is a daily chore akin to taking out the trash. If we take a day or three off from this task because we come down with a head cold or go on vacation, we come back to an inbox so cluttered with junk this daily chore becomes a cumbersome task.

The same holds true with most web pages. They all look the same.

Don't believe me? Check for yourself. Search out your competitors if you haven't already. Their websites mostly say the same thing... "We proudly serve our community," "Our doctors are the best," "We love helping our patients," We've been in business for 100 years." It's a cookie-cutter stamp they all share. The practice name may change, but the message is almost identical.

The internet and digital communication have morphed into an inflated and misused source of too much

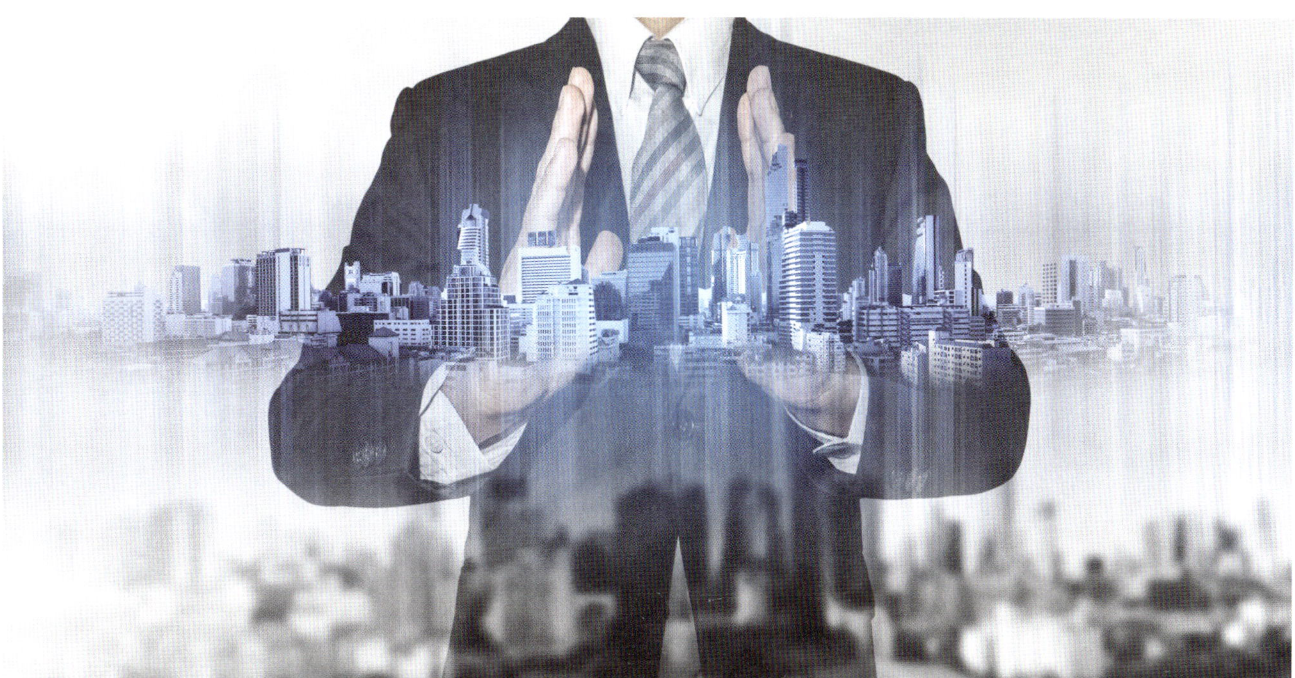

information mixed in with plenty of misinformation. This doesn't mean it's not important, but if you wish to have a compelling digital presence that connects with your patients, you must show up in a different light. The cookie-cutter approach simply will not do.

The good news is you can, and I'm about to show you how.

In this chapter, we'll discuss how to create a digital empire—a powerhouse, if you will, that connects with your patients and prospects in a meaningful way. We'll discuss how to craft and present compelling content online and through email that grabs and holds your readers' attention and makes them interested in what you offer and eager to accept treatment.

> *"Great design is the difference between lackluster and outstanding results."*
>
> – Parthiv Shah

LET'S START WITH YOUR WEBSITE, YOUR PIXEL ESTATE

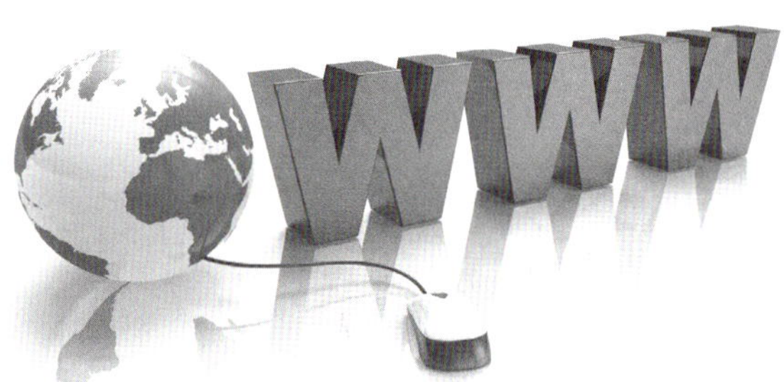

Your brick-and-mortar building where you practice dentistry is your real estate, and your web presence where you connect with your prospects and patients is your pixel estate—your place of doing business on the internet. Despite all the online digital noise, the internet is still where most of us seek out products and services. The problem for service providers and vendors is cutting through all that noise and connecting with prospects and patients.

Your Pixel Estate is the first thing your prospects see before interacting with you. And given how many cookie-cutter websites are out there, it's more important than ever that yours stands out. Your pixel estate must be designed and executed to appeal to your prospects' needs and wants, reduce apprehensions, and guide them through the buyer's journey. It must be visually, structurally and functionally sound to convert prospects into patients.

I call a website that meets these criteria a growth-driven design, or GDD website. Your GDD pixel estate must capture your values and personality so your audience grows to know, like and trust you and your practice. Your GDD pixel estate is fluid, changing sometimes from month to month based on data-driven results and decisions.

This means you must track which parts of your website generate the most business and maximize those targeted areas.

Over time and with your collected data, you'll understand your prospective patients' needs and wants and be able to serve them better by creating individualized patient journeys.

On all pages of your website, you want to address your patients' and prospects' needs and wants.

The backbone of your pixel estate is where your data lives. This is called your data warehouse or data cube. When your prospects enter your website, you want them under surveillance. You want to see where they spend their time, how long they scroll, what links they follow, and how long they remain on each page. This information will help you craft a compelling web presence, effective funnels, and email campaigns that connect with your current patients and help persuade prospects.

Now, let's talk about web pages that attract prospects and convert them into patients.

IF YOU WANT YOUR WEBSITE TO WORK FOR YOU AND DRAW IN YOUR IDEAL PROSPECTS, IT NEEDS TO HAVE THE FOLLOWING KEY PAGES:

- Home Page
- Cold Page
- Warm Page
- Hot Page
- Landing Page

Other pages, including a contact page and a testimonial page, can and probably should be added. But, for the most part, contact and testimonial pages write themselves.

Each website page needs to work toward maximizing your desired business results and fit with your overall marketing strategy. A website page that maximizes your results is called an optimized page or simply a page that sells.

TO OPTIMIZE EACH PAGE, YOU MUST FIRST ASK YOURSELF:

- What do my ideal prospects want?
- What problem drove them to look for a solution on your website?
- What information are they seeking as a solution to their problem?
- How can you give them the information they need so they trust you and see you as the source they seek to solve their problems?

Once you know what they want, you can deliver the information they need in an easily digestible format, such as a video, diagram or report.

Your optimization techniques for all your pages should:

1. Have a large, attention-grabbing headline that zeroes in on your patients' problems directly and clearly.

   Example headlines include:

   Are You Tired of Hating Your Smile?

   Would You Like to Look 10 Years Younger Without a Facelift?

   Do You Hate Your Dentures and Wish You Could Throw Them Away for Good?
2. Provide a logical flow of information that addresses patient issues and tells them exactly what to do next with your call to action (CTA).
3. A CTA that is obvious, direct and impossible to miss.
4. Important information displayed in the top portion of the web page.
5. Several CTAs on each page.
6. CTAs that allow your patients to easily contact you to schedule an appointment.
7. Website pages that focus on your patients' problems and how they can immediately resolve them with the treatment you provide.

Your optimized pages must address what your users want, deliver precisely that, and ask them to act in return.

Let's Start With Your Home Page

Your home page is a critical tool that acts as your practice's first impression. An in-person first impression takes 7 seconds. Your home page only has 3 seconds to make an excellent first impression. In those 3 seconds, you must introduce what you offer and compel your prospects to explore your site or download your resources. Your home page is the lead magnet that sets the stage for the conversation you wish to have with your prospects and the sales process you wish them to follow.

There are 14 key content features vital to your home page's success:

1. **Logo and headline:** It takes 2.6 seconds for a user's eye to land on the area of a website that most influences their first impression, your headline. And 46% of consumers base their decisions on the credibility of the website's visual appeal and esthetics. So, for your branding to make an impact, it should be front and center on the top of your website. Aim for a clear, simple headline that allows your ideal prospects to understand exactly what you offer within seconds.
2. **Sub-headline:** A user spends an average of 5.59 seconds looking at a website's written content. Your sub-headline should complement your headline and provide teaser information about what you offer while targeting a pain point in the process.
3. **Calls to Action (CTAs):** You want your visitors to quickly or eventually agree to the dental implants or treatment you offer. You want your CTAs to be prominent and easily accessible. They need to direct your prospects to different stages of your funnel. Link your CTAs to a landing page, a hot page, a cold page and a warm page. Make sure there is plenty of white space so the scanning eye easily finds them. They need to be short, five words or less preferably, and highly action oriented.
4. **Image or video:** An image or video of a handsome man or lovely woman with a confident smile or a video of someone discussing their before and after results can get your message across quickly and simply while adding interest and emotion to your page. You're

looking to capture the feeling and add integrity and believability here.

5. **Benefits:** Your prospects need to know the impact implants will have on their life. They need to understand the advantages of boosted confidence, how they will be perceived as younger and more attractive, and how their lives may be changed for the better if they only say yes to the treatment you recommend.
6. **Proof:** Testimonials are a great way to offer proof. Sprinkle them in. Add a few to your home page and anywhere else they make sense.
7. **Navigation route:** First impressions are 94% design related. This means if your website is too complicated or busy and navigation is not easy to understand, you'll lose most of your audience most of the time. Straightforward navigation that's visible on top of your page will make it easy and quick for your prospects to find what they're looking for.
8. **Content offer:** Gifting excellent free resources such as your ebook, blogs or special reports demonstrates your knowledge and credibility and encourages your prospects along the path by helping them solve their problems.
9. **Secondary CTAs:** These are in place to capture prospects who were not instantly interested in downloading a report or setting an appointment. They offer additional information and more reasons someone should seek out what you offer.
10. **List features:** The dental implants and high-value treatment you offer are unique, if for no other reason than it's you who offers them. Be sure to discuss what sets your practice and the treatment your prospects receive apart from the rest. Be concise and keep it easy to read.
11. **Resources:** Free resources are a great way to keep your visitors on your site longer and establish your trustworthiness as an expert.
12. **Awards and recognitions:** If you've won an award, received a special accommodation, or stood out as a shining star anywhere, this is where you legitimately brag about your accomplishments. In this setting, you're helping to establish your authority as an industry expert.
13. **Optimized for mobile devices.** The size of the population who use their phones as personal substitutes for personal computers grows higher each year. Smartphone searches are responsible for more than 60% of all website visits. This means it just makes sense to be sure your website is optimized for PCs and mobile devices.
14. **Information footer:** Once visitors reach the bottom of your page, they will want one or all of three things: Your contact information, a link to interior pages, or links to your social media. Be sure to offer all three in your footer.

A compelling home page makes it clear your site, which your prospects might have come across by searching a term like "dental implants" or "permanent tooth replacement," is precisely where they need to be. You want them to see that while yes you do provide quality options for tooth replacement, you also offer educational content that informs them of their treatment options and helps them decide what option is most likely to help them achieve their desired results.

Right from the start, you want to get into your ideal patient's head and address the questions going on there. You can do this with Call to Action (CTA) buttons that tease information that addresses those questions.

Your CTAs might be something like:

"Ready To Replace Missing Teeth?"

"What Happens if You Do Nothing?"

"Which Option is Right for You?"

Having several places on your home page where your prospect can say, "why yes, I would like to know more about my treatment options; I think I will click here, thank you very much," is an effective way to keep them engaged by speaking to the questions they already had stewing around in the back of their minds.

The Cold Page

Your cold page is where prospects land searching for information. It's your job to take problems they may be unaware of and make them aware of the pain points and consequences. Sure, your patients know they are missing teeth, but they may not know the problems with bone lurking just around the corner, waiting to wreak havoc on their facial structure if they do not permanently replace those missing teeth.

You must show them these pain points and how your dental implants solve these problems. While this is happening, you need to establish trust and credibility. Someone visiting your cold page may be only somewhat aware they need dental implants. They may still be considering dentures, bridges or doing nothing at all. Your job on your cold page is to answer their questions and nurture and educate them. A CTA on a cold page might be a button they can follow for a free report on the importance of replacing missing, damaged or decayed teeth.

Moving from a Cold Page to a Warm Page

The purpose of your warm page is to answer objections. And with dental implants, the biggest objection is typically the cost involved. On your warm page, you want to address this objection along with any others and make it clear that while dental implants have a hefty price tag upfront, there are several financing options available that make it affordable; their insurance may pay for some or most of the procedure, and even if they are uninsured, the value and benefits they will receive by replacing their damaged, decayed or missing teeth far out weight the initial upfront cost.

Your warm page is also a place to sift out those who can't afford dental implants. This way, you do not have to commit additional time and resources to a patient who, for financial reasons, will inevitably be forced to say no.

Converting Warm to Hot Pages

Once you've discussed your prospects' challenges and pain points and covered their objectives, it's time to convert them into patients by showing them the value they will receive by agreeing to the dental implants you offer. During the close, which happens on the hot page, there are only two predictable outcomes: your prospects say yes, and contact you ready to start treatment, or they say no thank you, go elsewhere, or choose to do nothing at all.

Your hot page is used to address prospects who know they have a problem, like missing or damaged teeth. They know dental implants are the only permanent solution. They know the cost of saying yes and understand what happens if they say no.

Your hot page needs to follow the **PADS** marketing approach. **Problem–Agitate—Discredit—Solve**. Identify the problem. Agitate the issue. Discredit alternate solutions. Solve the problem.

It should look something like this:

> "You know you're missing teeth, and your remaining teeth are decaying quickly. You know how painful it is to eat the foods you love and how you hate seeing your reflection in the mirror because of the state of your mouth and teeth. These problems are only what you see on the surface; the real problem is what's happening internally. How your jawbone is deteriorating, and how you're putting your whole system at risk by not properly addressing these gaping holes in your mouth. You could consider dentures, but they won't do anything to preserve your bone. You could get your dental implants somewhere that may be a few dollars cheaper, but do you really want to trust something so intricate and important to a discount dentist? Of course not. You want the most qualified professional to handle your dental implants at a reasonable price, and you want to love your results. Fortunately, you are in the right place. Click below to schedule your treatment."

When you identify the problem, you work to convince your prospects you have a deep understanding of their problem. When you agitate that problem, you get inside their head and scratch at what keeps them up at night and creates knots in their stomach during the day. Keep digging until you hit the source of their wound, then pour lemon juice on it. Be sure to point out the consequences they may not have known exist if they decline what you offer.

Are you worried your disfigured smile may cost you your next promotion?
Are you being shunned by the opposite sex because they can't stand your hideous smile?
Are you risking your health and possibly even your life by not fixing the rotten state of your mouth?

Next, discredit alternate solutions.

Dentures are no good, and discount dentists won't get you the results you're looking for.

Strike down alternatives one by one, take away all but a glimmer of hope...

Then, sweep in, like a knight in shining armor, and save the day.

Fortunately, the solution you need has been here all along.

Lead Magnet and Landing Page

A lead magnet is a marketing tool that helps you gain prospects' contact information in exchange for valuable content that helps them solve or, at least, understand their problems. A good lead magnet attracts their attention. When they click on your CTA button, they are taken to a landing page, a standalone web page on your website that is created to market toward a single focus or goal. On this landing page, your prospects can download your free report, request a free copy of your eBook, or set an appointment for a free smile consultation in your office. Your landing page should act as a hard-working conversion generator that reduces the time and cost of patient acquisition.

There are basically two types of landing pages:

Lead producing landing pages that use a form to collect names and emails.

Click-through landing pages that drive prospects straight to the appointment or sales page.

Your lead magnet needs to follow a step-by-step sales conversion trail starting with a compelling CTA button on your home page.

Once prospects click on your CTA, they are directed to your landing page. This page is an opportunity for you to connect and engage with your ideal prospects.

So, remember (PADS) Pain—Agitate—Solve—Discredit—Solve.

And showcase testimonials from satisfied, smiling patients. Most importantly, have a place where they enter their information—name, address, phone number and email—to receive your free content.

Once they hit submit, direct them to a simple thank you page that lets them know they have successfully submitted their information and will receive what you promised.

For a bonus, set up automated emails that send a message to your prospects, either with the digital information you promised or with the assurance they will receive it soon.

Leveraging YouTube Ads for Website Traffic

YouTube is a powerful platform for advertising due to its vast user base. You can connect with your ideal prospects by creating engaging and informative video content. This can include testimonials, or maybe you can briefly explain advancements in implant dentistry. The goal is to encourage your viewers to visit your website or landing page for more information.

You can use YouTube's advertising tools to target your ideal prospects, emphasizing demographics, their interest, or keywords they search for. This ensures your ads are seen by the audience most likely to be interested in what you offer. Include a clear and compelling call to action in your video and video description. Encourage viewers to visit your website, go to your landing page, or call your office for an appointment.

Harnessing Facebook and Social Media Platforms

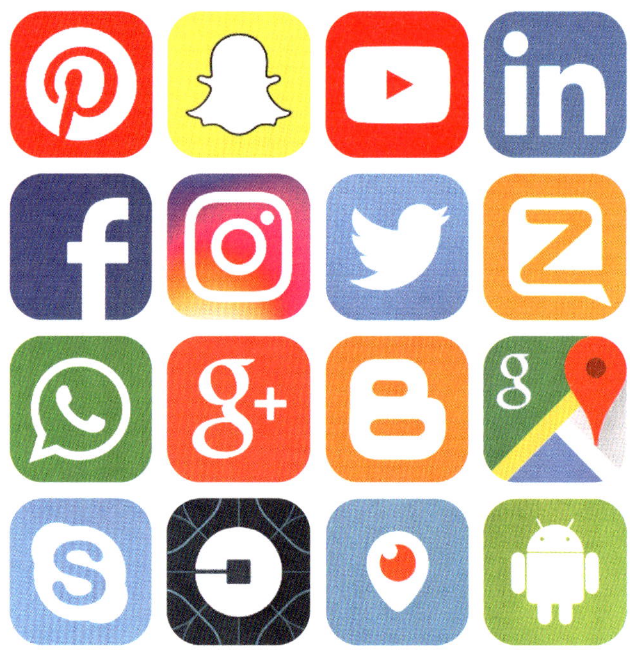

Facebook offers a robust advertising platform. Use visually appealing images or videos of smiling, satisfied patients, target your desired demographics, and use Facebook Pixel to track and retarget.

Regularly share engaging content on your social media channels. Encourage followers to share, like and comment, increasing the visibility of your posts and, consequently, your website.

Host contests or giveaways that require participants to visit your website. This not only boosts traffic but also increases awareness of your practice.

Geofencing for Targeted Marketing

Geofencing involves setting up a virtual perimeter around your location. You can use geofencing to send targeted ads to users' devices when they enter a predefined geographical area. This is particularly useful for attracting nearby customers. With Geofencing, you can send personalized offers or promotions to users within your geofenced area, encouraging them to visit your website for exclusive deals.

Understanding Search Engines and Organic vs. Paid Search

Optimize your website for search engines through on-page and off-page SEO techniques such as peppering your page with keywords, providing excellent and informative content, and backlinking to other websites. This helps improve organic search rankings, making your site more visible to the users you wish to attract.

Use paid search advertising, such as Google Ads, to appear at the top of search engine results for specific keywords such as "dental implants," "replace missing teeth," or "permanent solution to missing teeth." This provides immediate visibility and can complement your organic search efforts.

Workbook

Your Digital Empire Part I Workbook

Craft and present compelling content online and through email that grabs and holds your readers' attention and makes them interested in what you offer and eager to accept treatment. This workbook will help you create compelling web pages that resonate with your prospects. For more examples of successful pixel estate pages, please see the chapter on Samples and Swipe Files.

CREATING YOUR PIXEL ESTATE

Your pixel estate is your online storefront where your prospects and patients go to do business with you. If you want your website to work for you and draw in your ideal prospects, it needs to have the following key pages:

- Home Page
- Cold Page
- Warm Page
- Hot Page
- Landing Page

To optimize each page, first ask:

- What does my ideal prospects want?
- What problem drove them to look for a solution on your website?
- What information are they seeking as a solution to their problem?
- How can you give them the information they need so they trust you and see you as the source they seek to solve their problems?

Each page must have:

- A compelling headline
- A Call to Action (CTA)
- Important information your readers need to know
- Additional CTAs at various places on each page that go to a place where prospects can contact you or schedule an appointment.
- Content that focuses on your patients' problems and how they can immediately resolve them with the treatment you recommend.

Your Home Page: Your Practice's First Impression

There are 14 key content features vital to your home page's success:

1. **Logo and headline**: Aim for a clear, simple headline that, in a few seconds, clearly defines what you offer and what you are about.

2. **Sub-headline:** Your sub-headline should complement your headline and provide teaser information about your offer while targeting a pain point.

3. **Calls to Action (CTAs):** You want your visitors to quickly or eventually agree to the dental implants or treatment you offer. You want your CTAs to be prominent and easily accessible. They need to be short, five words or less preferably, and highly action oriented.

4. **Image or video:** An image or video of a handsome man or lovely woman with a confident smile or someone discussing before-and-after results. Do you already have this content? Who can you use to produce this video?

5. **Benefits:** Your prospects need to know how implants or the treatment you recommend will benefit their lives. What benefits would you like to highlight for the treatment you recommend?

6. **Proof:** Testimonials are a great way to offer proof. Sprinkle them in. Which case studies or customer reviews would you like to highlight on your home page?

7. **Content offer:** What is your irresistible offer for prospects visiting your home page?

8. **Secondary CTAs:** These are in place to capture prospects who were not instantly interested in downloading a report or setting an appointment. They offer additional information and more reasons someone should seek out what you offer. What valuable content might you add to keep your prospects engaged?

9. **List features:** The dental implants and high-value treatment you offer are unique, if for no other reason than it's you who offers them. What sets you apart as a dental authority? Why should your prospects drive past competitors and insist you are the only one they allow to touch their teeth? Be concise and keep it easy to read.

10. **Resources:** Free resources are a great way to keep your visitors on your site longer and establish your trustworthiness as an expert. What valuable free resources and content can you offer your prospects?

11. **Awards and recognitions:** You want to establish your authority by discussing what sets you apart. Discuss your education, awards and features on podcasts, TV, or as a keynote speaker. What have you done that you want to be sure your patients are aware of?

Workbook

12. **Cold Page**

What problems might prospective patients face without their awareness? Use your cold page to discuss these problems and identify the pain points and consequences.
Here's an example: If patients are missing teeth, they might be aware they have problems chewing or hate the way the missing tooth looks in their mouth, but they may not be aware of the risk they are of degenerative changes to their jawbone and facial structure.
Start with a catchy headline and establish trust and credibility. Your job is to offer valuable information and answer questions you know prospects might ask. The CTA on a cold page might allow them to download a free special report on the subjects you cover. Brainstorm some ideas for the content you might add on your cold page:

13. **Warm Page**

The purpose of your warm page is to answer objections. This often means discussing costs or the need for what some might consider invasive surgery.
A good way of addressing this is to discuss cost/benefit objectives and the true cost of doing nothing and suffering the consequences. Be sure to have a good headline. The CTA for this page might be to schedule a free consultation to learn more.
What objections do you commonly hear from your patients? Spend some time jotting them down and your answers in response to these objections:

14. **Hot Page**

This is where you convert prospects into patients by showing them the value they will receive by agreeing to the treatment you recommend.
Your hot page needs to Identify the problem. Agitate the issue. Discredit alternate solutions. Solve the problem. Refer back to the conversation in Chapter 8 about the PADS technique, then spend a few moments brainstorming on the topics you would like to cover on your hot page:

Workbook

Chapter 9
Your Digital Empire Part II

We've discussed building your pixel estate and all that entails, but there's more to your digital empire than just your website.

How can you leverage effective funnels, lead captures and landing pages to get your prospects saying YES before they even step foot through your door?

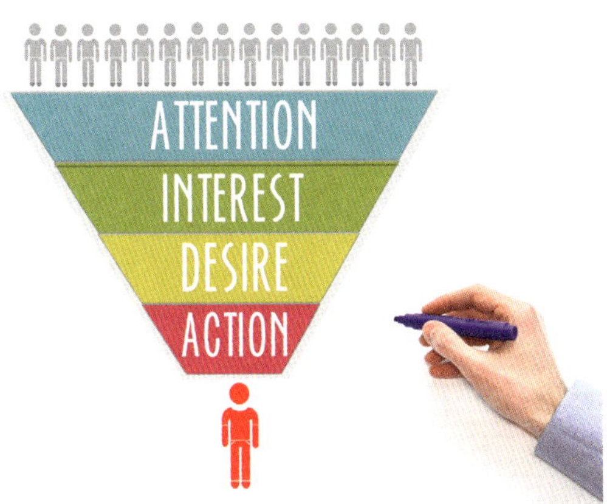

The first part of an effective funnel is your CTA.

Whether your prospect finds you with a Google search, on a YouTube video, or a blog post, you want your CTA to be engaging.

HERE ARE SOME EXAMPLES OF CTAS THAT GRAB ATTENTION:

1. **Get My Free ebook on Advancements in Dental Implants.**
2. **Download Your Guide to Permanent Tooth Replacement.**
3. **Unlock the Secrets of the Hollywood Smile.**

The trick is to be creative and genuine. You have content that will benefit your ideal prospects. You know it, and they need to know it as well.

THE OFFER PAGE/AKA THE LANDING PAGE

Offer pages are known by many names, including landing pages, lead capture pages, single property pages, static pages, squeeze pages, and destination pages. These monikers are all used to describe a page on your website that displays directed sales copy.

A website with a landing page, or maybe two or three, offers additional opportunities to turn your visitors into your patients.

The purpose of a landing page is to act as the top of your funnel through a sales campaign that targets a specific group with a special promotion. You want to promote implants or your high-value service by pinpointing a specific problem, such as how missing teeth can make it hard to smile in public or how dentures are uncomfortable to wear and are a potential source of embarrassment. Then, offer a solution in the form of a downloadable book, special report, or free in-office smile consultation.

Your page should feature a clickable button that sends visitors to the next stage of the sales process. If they say yes to the free report, the next stage may be a squeeze page asking for more information to mail them a hard copy. If they say yes to the smile consultation, the next stage may be a thank you page informing them someone will call to schedule their appointment.

If you give your prospects too many options and too many places to go, they may get confused or overwhelmed and freeze. Some people call this analysis paralysis. Instead, make your offer clear and concise. This is why your landing page is a singular event. Your offer page should only make one offer with one clickable button that takes visitors to a single location.

Make sure your offer teases valuable content, is straightforward, and is easy to say yes to. And make sure you're tracking your results. If your offer is not generating sales every month, then there's room for improvement. Be prepared to make changes and experiment with different landing pages to achieve the best results.

I recommend having multiple offer pages. This will show you which topics are the most popular and which convert the most leads. Pay attention to these metrics and you will better understand your audience and know where to focus your efforts.

THE ASK FUNNEL

This is a highly effective way to get to know your prospects.

The ask funnel is a formula that gets your prospects to engage with you in a way that's meaningful to them. In this funnel, you simply ask them, "Do you have a specific question?" Be sure to include valuable content on this page as well; this may be a good place for a FAQ with a few broad questions that may give prospects some of the answers they seek. But the main reason for this page is to get them to provide their name, email address, phone number, and the question that's weighing on their mind. Imagine how easy it would be to connect meaningfully with your ideal prospects if you knew precisely what interested them or kept them up at night. This is the power of the ask funnel.

THE REFERRAL PAGE

This page can help you turn your ideal patients into raving fans and your best recruiters.

Referrals are solid gold because people buy from people they trust. Turning general practitioners, family dentists, mothers, fathers, neighbors, sisters, and brothers into recruiters is a phenomenally effective way to bring in new business to your practice. Having a place where satisfied patients can refer their friends or family is a smart move that, when executed correctly, will drive business to your practice.

SQUEEZE PAGES

If prospects have said yes once, they will likely say yes to more.

A squeeze page is a way to capture additional information and market to your prospects.

In 2023, it was estimated that approximately 300 billion emails were sent worldwide every day. I'm sure you received your fair share of these emails and met them with the same enthusiastic morning, afternoon or evening inbox purge that's so common to us all.

This is why a second squeeze page is so important. After prospects agree to download your free report, hit them again with a winning offer. "Would you prefer a hard copy of this report be delivered to your front door? All you need to do is provide your address, and we'll ship one immediately." Now, you not only have their email but also their physical address. This means you can market to them with targeted postcards and sales letters. Equally important, you've captured valuable data that may pinpoint a hotspot in the community where you can direct marketing efforts in the future. Bottom line: Squeeze pages are effective, which helps ring the cash register.

THE PILLAR PAGE

A pillar page is like a landing page that covers all aspects of a topic in-depth and then links to clusters or pillars of related content. To create your pillar page, consider your ideal prospects—their problems, challenges and interests—and choose a topic that speaks to that. Your pillar page could include a long-form post on oral health and how it relates to overall physical and mental health. You could hyperlink to a cluster of topics, including advancements in dental implants or the perils of periodontal disease. Each hyperlink offers a deep dive into its specific topic. As prospects read through your pillar page, they can jump to specific topics they want to learn more about. A bonus: Search engines LOVE these cluster models, and they will help you maintain a higher ranking without spending a dime on optimization.

LONG-TERM NURTURE

An effective way to build top-of-the-mind awareness is through targeted email.

A long-term nurture (LTN) email campaign can be a highly effective strategy for engaging prospective patients, building trust, offering valuable content, addressing concerns, showcasing your expertise, highlighting your success stories, and guiding your prospects toward considering high-value dental treatment and dental implants.

A weekly email campaign allows you to gradually build trust and establish a relationship with your prospective patients. You create credibility and reliability by consistently providing valuable information, addressing common concerns related to dental implants, and sharing success stories or testimonials. Over time, this fosters a connection between your dental practice and prospective patients.

A key advantage of an LTN campaign is the opportunity to deliver educational content. Use the weekly emails to share insights about the benefits of dental implants, the implant procedure and aftercare, and address any misconceptions or fears. Providing informative content showcases your expertise and empowers patients to make informed decisions about their dental health.

Prospective patients often have questions and concerns about dental procedures, especially those perceived as high value like dental implants. A well-crafted email campaign allows you to address these concerns systematically. Each week, focus on a specific aspect, whether it's the procedure's safety, the durability of implants, or the recovery process. Proactively addressing these concerns alleviates doubts and builds confidence in your practice.

Highlighting your dental practice's expertise and success stories is crucial in persuading prospective patients. Share case studies, before-and-after photos, or testimonials in your emails. Personal narratives from patients who have undergone successful dental implant treatments can be particularly compelling, serving as real-world examples of the positive outcomes your practice can deliver.

Each email should include a clear call to action that guides prospective patients toward the next step. Whether it's scheduling a free smile consultation or accessing exclusive resources on your website, the CTA should encourage engagement.

By consistently providing valuable content, addressing concerns, and strategically guiding prospective patients through decision-making, you increase the likelihood of converting leads into patients interested in high-value treatments like dental implants.

AUTOMATED EMAILS

Use these tools to persuade potential patients to set appointments and commit to treatment.

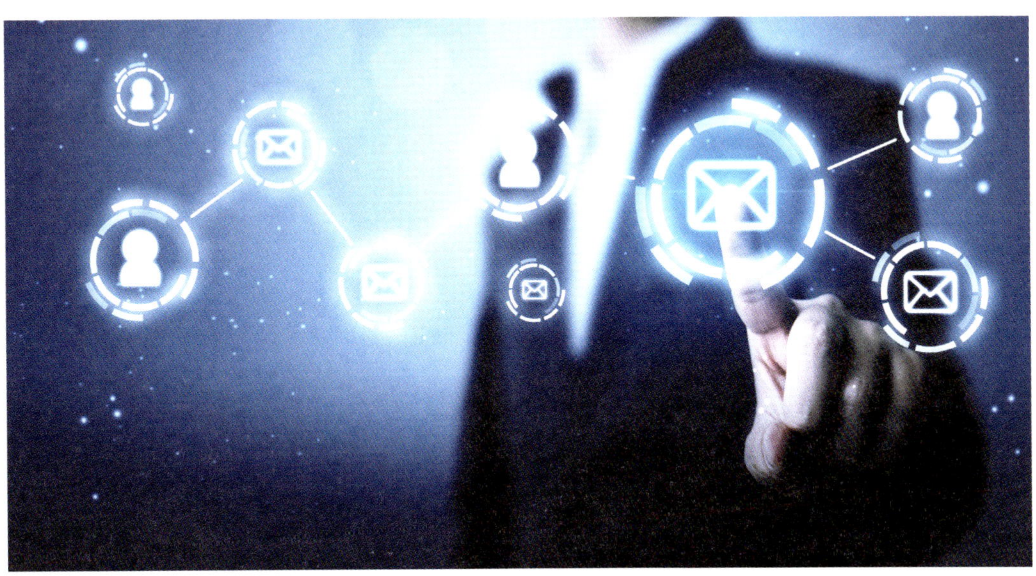

Examples include:

New lead emails. These emails provide an excellent opportunity to introduce new leads to dental implants and other high-end dental services your practice offers. These emails can provide a brief overview of the benefits of dental implants, address common concerns, and emphasize the expertise and advanced technology available at your dental practice.

They also can serve as educational tools, delivering valuable content to help leads make informed decisions about their dental health. Provide insights into the advantages of dental implants, the implantation process, and the potential impact on oral well-being. By offering educational content, you position your practice as a trusted source of information and support.

New lead emails can include exclusive offers or incentives to encourage leads to take the next step. This could involve a free smile consultation or access to your special report on dental implants. Providing tangible benefits creates a sense of value and urgency, which motivates leads to engage with your practice.

Be sure to include a clear CTA to schedule a consultation or follow a link for downloadable content. Make it easy for prospects to take the next step.

With this consistent communication, you become familiar with and build trust with your prospects. Share information about your practice's values, the expertise of your dental professionals, and the positive experiences of other patients. Trust is a critical factor in the decision-making process for high-end dental services, and these emails contribute to establishing a solid foundation for a long-term patient-practitioner relationship.

By combining informative content, special offers, and personalized communication, these emails build a relationship with potential patients and encourage them to take the next step toward optimal oral health.

New patient welcome sequences. These emails help new patients feel at home with your practice.

The welcome sequence sets the tone for a positive onboarding experience for new dental implant patients. These initial emails can express enthusiasm for their decision to choose your practice, provide essential information about what to expect during the implant procedure, and assure them of the expert care they will receive.

The sequence can be designed to provide a step-by-step overview of the dental implant process. This includes pre-procedural preparations, implantation day, and post-procedure care instructions. This information helps manage patient expectations and empowers them with knowledge, reducing any anxieties they might have.

The welcome sequence also can be a practical tool for coordinating logistics. Provide clear instructions for appointment scheduling, details about necessary paperwork or pre-surgical requirements, and contact information for any queries related to the upcoming dental implant procedure. Smooth coordination contributes to a positive patient experience.

Appointment no-show emails. Use these emails to reengage patients who missed appointments. By reaching out promptly after the missed appointment, you demonstrate your practice's commitment to their care and emphasize the importance of their dental health.

Include options for rescheduling the missed appointment or booking a new one. Provide a convenient way for patients to rectify the situation, such as online scheduling or a dedicated phone number.

Even after a missed appointment, regular communication helps strengthen the patient-provider relationship. It shows your practice cares about their well-being and will work with them to ensure they receive necessary care. This positive communication can contribute to patient loyalty. Addressing missed appointments strategically can improve patient communication, reduce revenue loss, and enhance the overall patient experience.

Appointment no-sale email sequences. These emails are crucial for engaging patients who attended a dental implant consultation but did not immediately commit to treatment.

Patients may not be ready to make immediate decisions about dental implant treatment during the initial consultation. An appointment no-sale email sequence allows you to continue the conversation, providing additional information, addressing concerns, and nurturing the relationship over time. This ongoing engagement may eventually guide your patients toward a confident decision.

Use the email sequence as an educational tool. Provide in-depth information about the benefits of dental implants, the procedure itself, and the long-term advantages for oral health. Offer valuable content in a structured sequence. This way, you contribute to your patients' understanding and help them make an informed decision when they feel ready.

Consistent communication through the email sequences help build trust and confidence. Once again, share success stories from other patients who have undergone dental implant procedures at your practice. Testimonials and before-and-after photos can provide tangible evidence of your dental professionals' positive outcomes and expertise.

Patients may have lingering concerns or questions following the initial consultation. Use these emails to address these concerns systematically. Encourage patients to ask questions and proactively address common concerns about the dental implant procedure, recovery and aftercare.

In the email sequence, incorporate incentives or special offers to encourage patients to proceed with their dental implant treatment. This could include exclusive discounts, complimentary services, or additional perks for scheduling their procedure within a specified timeframe.

Satisfaction surveys and referral requests. This is how you turn satisfied patients into raving fans.

Implementing a series of emails that begins with a customer satisfaction survey about the dental implant procedure and concludes with a referral request can be a great way to gain insight into the patient experience and drum up business for your practice.

Start this email sequence with a customer satisfaction survey. This allows you to gauge your patients' overall satisfaction with their dental implant procedure. Understanding their experience, including aspects like quality of care, communication, and post-operative support, provides valuable insights into areas of strength and areas that may need improvement.

If the survey indicates concerns or areas where patients felt less satisfied, subsequent emails in the series can be strategically designed to address these issues. This proactive approach demonstrates a commitment to continuous improvement and patient-centric care, fostering a sense of trust and loyalty.

Express genuine interest in your patients' well-being. You strengthen your connection with your patients this way and enhance the likelihood of ongoing engagement and loyalty.

As the series progresses, and if your patients express satisfaction with their dental implant procedure, the final emails can introduce the idea of referrals. Happy and satisfied patients often recommend you to friends, family or colleagues. By including a referral request at the conclusion of the series, a successful dental implant procedure, coupled with a positive post-operative experience, can turn patients into advocates for your practice.

AN UNSTOPPABLE FORCE

Well, there you have it, folks. If you weren't convinced of the power and effectiveness of a well-crafted digital empire before, I hope you are now. When combined with a powerful direct mail presence, you turn your marketing efforts into an unstoppable force that will aid in new patient acquisition, patient retention, and re-engaging old patients.

The chapters on the power of print assets and creating your digital empire are the heart and soul of this book. Still, we have more to cover. They don't call me Mr. Implementation for nothing. Stay tuned because we're about to discuss streamlining and automation and how it can be a game changer for your practice.

Chapter 10
Streamlining and Automating Your Internal Management Systems

Save time and money while ensuring your business is run according to your standards.

In this chapter, we will discuss:

1. Your marketing automation plan
2. Content and project management systems
3. Contact and customer relationship management systems
4. Opportunity management systems
5. Money and document management systems
6. User management systems
7. Learning management systems

If you've read this far and you're still with me, congratulations! There are a lot of steps and a lot of content. If you execute all of it and get it right, you can accelerate your practice at warp speed and be miles ahead of your competitors in no time. Still, it's a lot of work. That's why so many dentists I speak with decide to hire me. They focus on running their practice while I do the heavy lifting, developing and implementing all the assets we've covered so far.

I promised I'd cover it all, from soup to nuts, and this book would not be complete if we skipped what may be the most important part—and what makes all of this manageable—and that is streamlining and automating your management systems.

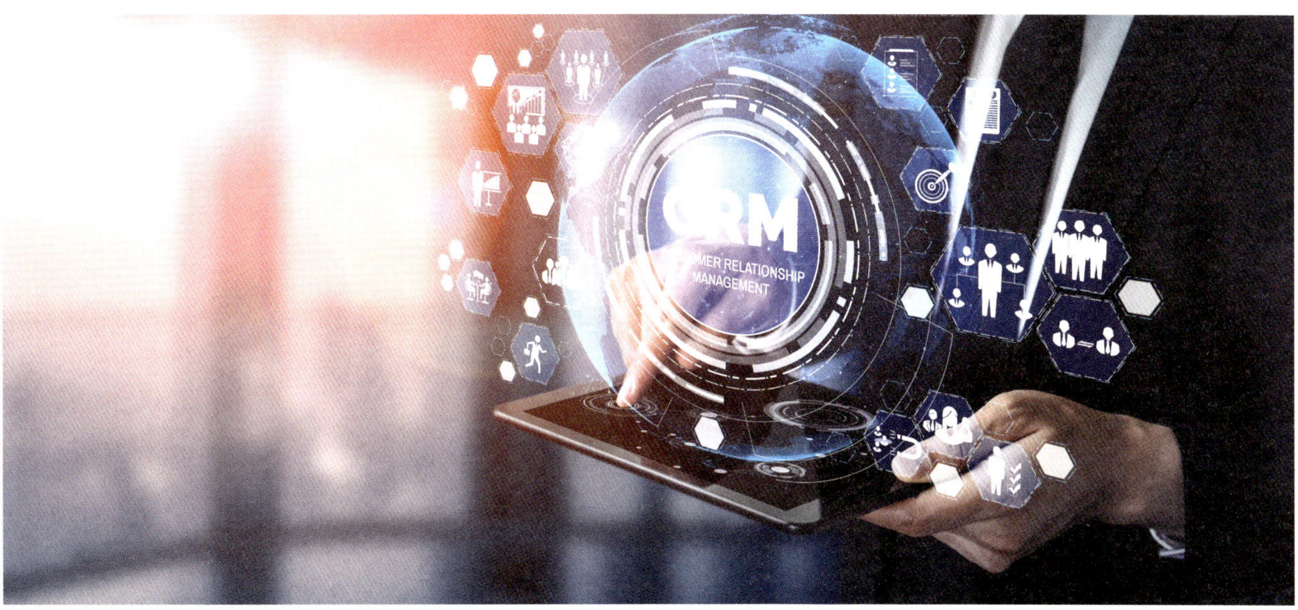

Let me start by saying that if you haven't already, I highly recommend investing in a CRM system that integrates with your website from day one. This type of system assimilates all the functionalities of your website and handles inbound and outbound marketing and sales. It helps convert leads into patients and can grow and expand your business as needed.

Otherwise, you're forced to handle all the marketing efforts we've discussed piecemeal, assigning staff and tying up personnel to track patients and connect with prospects. This can be cumbersome and draining, to say the least, and will likely result in missed opportunities and upset patients and team members.

An integrated system, on the other hand, puts your business in the right position from the beginning. This way, you and your staff work with effective marketing that collects information about your prospects from multiple channels, such as web page activity and social media, and builds an ongoing relationship. Implementing an integrated system helps you grow your business, build customer loyalty, and organize yourself and your business.

WITH AN INTEGRATED SYSTEM YOU CAN:

- Create and manage a constant crop of leads.
- Nurture your prospects with ease and automation.
- Track your patients' digital fingerprints across multiple channels, which helps you recognize and respond to their needs.
- Easily publish search engine-optimized and appealing blog content and landing pages.
- Create and distribute tailored emails with engaging content and subject lines.
- Gather analytics from your social media, SEO, CTAs, and any other online advertising you may implement.
- Synchronize your database to easily access emails, forms and segmented lists.

The CRM system I'm talking about exists; it's affordable, and it's how I help my clients attract more customers and convert more leads, resulting in a higher ROI than they ever imagined possible. If you'd like more information on how I make this happen for my clients, your next step is easy: go to www.meetparthiv.com and schedule a time to talk.

USING AUTOMATION AND DEVELOPING YOUR MARKETING AUTOMATION PLAN (MAP)

You have a database of patients and prospects and know who you want to market to and what type of message they should receive. Once you have your marketing message down, you can automate it using off-the-shelf marketing automation tools.

There are many marketing automation tools on the market, such as HubSpot, Keap (formerly Infusionsoft), ClickFunnels, GoHighLevel, ActiveCampaign, and many others. Personally, I prefer HubSpot and use it for my own business.

I have worked with numerous CRMs throughout my career, and my own creation, eBGS (eLaunchers Business GROWTH System), built on a HIPAA-compliant GoHighLevel platform, truly warms my heart.

First, when I was writing this book, it was the least expensive application in its class. For an initial set-up fee of about $2,000 and about$300 monthly, you have an application that can work as your marketing automation engine, primary data warehouse, and data intelligence system. eBGS: eLaunchers Best GROWTH System is a single database with multi-faceted functionalities. It creates a record of each client, prospect, referral, and staff member and keeps track of all touchpoints, including emotional and fiscal interactions. It is a single database with CRM functionality, marketing automation functionality, lead capture functionality, e-commerce functionality, sales force automation functionality, and an email marketing system all in one.

It integrates ALL communication channels, including email, direct mail, text messaging, and more. It tells your staff what needs to be done and reminds your patients of appointments. eBGS: eLaunchers Best GROWTH System is intuitive and user-friendly when compared to the alternatives. It is powerful, and of course, with power comes complexity. It may not be for the faint of heart, but if you are willing to invest the time, you can learn to use it without extensive training or a special certification.

Now, please understand you CAN implement this yourself. And if you look to the resources tab on my website, elaunchers.com, you'll find the campaign blueprint from my eBGS: eLaunchers Best GROWTH System. It's yours for the taking, a gift cheerfully given. You can implement the workflow yourself or hire a consultant to implement it for you.

I'd like to give you a taste of what this blueprint can do. It starts with:

1. **Lead generation.** This is where you will go through segmentation and approach to generate quality traffic to your website, home page, landing pages, etc. If you choose to build your website, you might use WordPress and leadpages.net or the Optimize Press plugin for WordPress to build landing pages, thank you, and referral pages. Be sure to add your squeeze pages as well. You want the initial squeeze to capture the name, email and phone number and the thank you page, which is a second squeeze, to capture the physical address and phone number so you can deliver a promised tangible gift such as a shock and awe package or special report.
2. **Lead conversion:** New lead follow-up sequences have three to five emails and at least two telephone follow-up steps. The purpose is to reiterate the landing page's message and persuade the prospect to schedule an appointment and discuss the next steps in the sales process.
3. **Long-term nurture.** This is a 24-month campaign that includes a monthly newsletter, weekly emails, holiday cards, and a twice-a-year gift. This is in addition to occasional special marketing efforts to convert an unconverted lead and lost opportunity. This might sound complex, but it will set you apart from your competitors and keep your name fresh in your prospects' minds.
4. **Appointment confirmation sequence.** Send out information about what an initial implant consultation entails, including directions to your office, rules of engagement, and what you're trying to accomplish. Set the groundwork so patients know what to expect when they arrive.
5. **Appointment prognosis sequence**. This consists of the appointment no-show, appointment no sale or sold and welcome to our practice emails. You should have an email, print and telephone sequence for each scenario as well, with the correct sequences triggered depending on the prognosis of the appointment.
6. **Satisfaction survey and tell a friend.** This is where you ask patients who have recently completed their implant procedure how they feel about their implants, and then, later in the email sequence, follow up with a request for a referral to someone they know who may benefit from implants as well.
7. **Patient long-term nurture:** Your patients also need a long-term nurture sequence. This campaign requires about a dozen web pages, copy for about three dozen email messages, telephone scripts, and a substantial amount of print material. If your revenue model doesn't justify printing expensive shock and awe packages plus books and the cost of FedEx boxes, send only a printed letter inviting patients to a URL where they can read more in digital format.

By developing a customized, unique and highly specialized marketing automation plan, you can design a "Perfect Customer Life Cycle" process. This set of interlinking, technology-enabled systems facilitates business growth, profitability and security more than anything else. Items like newsletters or e-zines allow you to stay in touch with those who've shown an interest but are not ready to buy.

You want to be seen not just as a dentist but as a dental implant specialist—a trusted source and authority on implant application and placement. Offering special reports, content-rich blog posts, video tutorials, webinars, ebooks, e-newsletters, and podcasts are ways to educate potential patients, connect with them, and build trust.

This system, once deployed, can help you capture leads, nurture prospects who are already in your pipeline, stay in touch with those who are not yet ready to say yes, persuade potential patients to agree to implants, and more.

Automated systems can help keep your current patients happy and encourage your former patients to refer their friends and family to you for their needed implants and dental treatment.

LET'S REVIEW THE STEPS YOU MUST TAKE IF YOU CHOOSE TO FLY SOLO:

1. Pick a target market that needs dental implants or high-end dental treatment.
2. Craft an irresistible free offer that pokes at your prospects' problems and then promises a solution with a special free report, ebook, or other value-added content.
3. Ideally, you would then use eBGS: eLaunchers Best GROWTH System to capture contact information, deliver the irresistible free offer, and follow up to take the next step.
4. Then, promote that offer to your target market.

If all this works, and your ideal patients click on your CTA in your Facebook ad, blog post, or home page, they say yes to the free report and possibly to the physical copy as well, then congratulations! Your process is in motion, and you've established trust with your prospects. Now comes the fun part. You need to get them to take the next step in your relationship:

THE NEXT STEP COULD BE:

- Opening your next email.
- Clicking on a link in the next email you send them.
- Using your website to book a free smile consultation.
- Setting and keeping an appointment.
- Or several other options depending on what you wish to accomplish—it's limited only by your imagination.

Now, I know what you're thinking. That's a lot of steps. And you're right. It is. But if you want to take your practice to the next level, this is a tried-and-true formula to get you there. So, your options are to hire me and let me manage this while you manage your practice, appoint someone on your staff to do it, or take your multitasking to an entirely new level.

Chapter 11
Can My System Work for a VERY SMALL Dental Practice?

The short answer is YES. The system as a whole CAN work for a very small dental practice... but the dentists who own them may or may not have the financial means to invest in the complete system. A practice making less than half a million dollars in revenue is unlikely to have the cash flow and cash reserves to make a six-figure investment in their growth.

The REAL challenge in helping a very small dental practice grow is the lack of data. They just don't have enough unconverted leads and lost opportunities in their dental patient database. They have diamonds in their dental database, but the diamond mine is very small.

So, when we can work with growth-minded, progressive dentists looking to grow their practice, we do things a little differently. We look for ways to implement small fractions of our complete system and use that to acquire growth. Once they grow, they invest in the rest of the system.

We all know there are three parts to a sales funnel: top of the funnel (TOFU); middle of the funnel (MOFU); and bottom of the funnel (BOFU).

When resources are tight, the budget is low, and there is not enough time to practice my trade, my strategy is to disregard TOFU and MOFU and focus on making the BOFU more productive. We start with improved case presentation material, better print experience for patients, and better patient education materials. This is likely to have a bigger impact faster.

Sometimes, the practice is struggling because there are just not enough new patients, new inquiries and new leads, AND there are not enough diamonds in the dental database to get desirable growth. In situations like this, we talk about "micro-campaigns" to develop relevant and targeted traffic that is likely to generate desired growth.

There is no one-size-fits-all traffic strategy. Dentistry commonly uses a cocktail of online and offline traffic, leveraging paid and organic marketing coupled with direct mail outreach. This strategy fails if you don't provide creative direction to your traffic sources.

If your lead associate dentist wants to sell teeth straightening, you want to target young, affluent households. SOMEONE needs to have this conversation with the practice owner, associate doctors, and the traffic companies who do SEO, PPC, social media posting, Facebook or Instagram ads, and direct mail postcards. SOMEONE needs to be in charge of deciding WHO we are marketing to and WHAT we are going to offer this week, this month, this quarter.

Lack of money and data are not the only issues in very small dental practices; there are other problems to consider. There is usually a lack of standardized systems and processes. To make matters worse, the doctor is not the best salesperson, the staff lacks a sales mindset, and there is nearly zero patient education material in place. The practice just "floats" into existence.

Working with these practices is most painful and difficult for a marketing agency. It's like putting shoes on Tarzan. Everything is done for the first time. Nothing makes sense. Everyone is skeptical, and no one except the lead doctor has bought into the business growth process.

When we work with practices like this, we don't try to teach their humans how to do sales or marketing. There are coaches and practice growth consultants who are suited to help dentists train their team. We don't do that. We create systems, processes and marketing assets that are deployed WITHOUT using the in-office staff.

Wrapping Up: How This Program Can Change Your Life

> *"The world you desire can be won. It exists…it is real…it is possible…it is yours."*
>
> *- Ayn Rand*

To you, my reader, the skilled dentist tired of spending long hours as a slave, chained to the dental chair...

I predict life-changing results if you implement the strategies and assets discussed in this book.

You know there's more to owning a dental practice than the demanding job and workload you're currently forced to manage.

You know you want more and you know others who've already accomplished what you want. If they can do it, you can too.

You want a business that works for you—a money-making machine that attracts high-dollar patients who enthusiastically agree to dental treatment and happily recommend their friends and family for dental treatment at your office.

The specific details and insider strategies I've provided in this book will take your dental practice from barely out of the red to achieving higher gross revenues than you may have dreamed possible.

The strategic guidance and automated marketing systems I've gone over have helped practice owners grow from a few hundred thousand in gross revenue to more than $2 million in less than 12 months. Others have taken their practices to more than $12 million in gross income in less than 18 months.

The strategies and assets I discussed in this book reveal the secrets of how they did it.

Many of these practice owners chose to hire me directly and let me do the heavy lifting while they focused on running their practice. You can do this too. If you are serious about growth, then give me a call. Let's discuss what we can do for your practice in the next 12 to 18 months.

This book is designed to help you at any stage of growth, whether you're just starting out and struggling to clear $100K a year or you're already making a million plus in gross revenue and looking to take your practice to a new level. Whether you chose to work with me or not, this book will help you achieve your greatest year yet.

A business with marketing strategies that deliver effective messages to the right market time and time again grows at an exponential pace. This book shows you how to implement these strategies in your practice and reach gross revenue that's two to five times higher than you achieved in any other year, all within the next 12 months or less.

With the right marketing strategies, patient education tools, and automated response systems in place, it is easy for a dental practice to attract higher-value patients, ease the workload for the dentist or practice owner, and keep patients lined up, presold and eager to start treatment.

In this book, I've identified the business growth strategies, direct marketing campaigns, and automated marketing response efforts that are TESTED and PROVEN to deliver higher gross revenue for dental practices just like yours.

If you are ready to change your dental practice and income forever, then reading, absorbing and implementing the proven strategies I've discussed in this book will guide you on your way.

Wishing you success in all that you do.

Sincerely,

Parthiv Shah

www.meetparthiv.com

Guest Chapter by Alice Pettey

Branding 101 for Dentists

Branding is not a subject that came up in dental school. Now that you are a successful dentist, you've discovered what was lacking in your education. There were many topics outside the clinical activities of dentistry that you now see would have helped prepare you to run your practice.

WHO AM I, AND WHY SHOULD YOU LISTEN TO ME?

My name is Alice Pettey; I hold a Master of Fine Arts in Media Design, focusing on developing comprehensive client branding. I have completed numerous branding courses, including Brand Master Academy and Level C Brand Specialist and Strategist certifications. I am certified as a Buyers Persona Expert, the author *of Branding Your Practice: A Comprehensive Guide to Building a Strong Brand in Health & Wellness*, and the founder and editor of "Differentiate Magazine," a quarterly publication directed at the branding and growth of health and wellness practices. I have worked in the branding and design industry since 1999 and with Parthiv Shah at eLauncher.com since 2012, providing him and his clients with various branding and design services.

Now that we've cleared up all the credentials, we can get down to what matters... branding your practice!

SETTING THE FOUNDATIONS

You may want to jump right in and pick some colors and a typeface (or font) and make a logo. But while an *Identity System* is part of your branding, it is not where you should start.

An identity system, as it relates to branding and design, provides direction and rules for a company's visual aspects. Many elements go into creating an identity system. These include the logo and stationery; colors; graphics; patterns; textures; the visual appearance of marketing collateral: brochures, direct mail, website design, email, social media, magazine, billboard, and display advertising; product design and packaging; uniforms; signage; and vehicle graphics.

These elements do not make up every company's identity system. Some have more, and some have less. An identity system needs to address the visual, tonal and all the company's potential visual impressions. Additionally, it must minimize inconsistent or nonexistent identity applications that result in non-optimal brand perception. With all these elements in play, developing a Standards document becomes paramount.

Well, then, where do you start?

I'm glad you asked! You start at the beginning. With "WHY"... Why are you in business? Why do you do what you do? Why do you work with the people you work with? Why do you serve the clients you serve?

I am going to take you on this journey with an actual client. Together, we will see the dentist's progression through the branding process, I also will guide you through the process of establishing a brand for your practice.

CASE STUDY: NORTH CAROLINA CENTERS FOR DENTAL EXCELLENCE

The Problem

Marcia Rementer, DMD, struggled with a growing practice and a fragmented visual brand. Dr. Rementer and

David (her husband and practice manager) wanted to produce a cohesive visual brand while providing visual cues (color) to each office location.

When they came to me, the conversation centered on their desire for a new logo. They felt the one they currently had was no longer serving them completely. In fact, they had taken on additional locations over the years, which had left them with a disjointed and fragmented image.

Patients needed clarification and help to connect each location to the whole practice, as each office had a look or feel independent of the others.

During our initial conversations, we explored who Dr. Rementer was and her vision for her practices. These conversations helped us discover the foundation that would make up the new brand standards for the North Carolina Centers for Dental Excellence.

We started with "why."

Why was Dr. Rementer in practice? She had a desire to help her patients have happier, more fulfilled lives by giving them the confidence that comes with a healthy, beautiful smile. She wanted to challenge the impersonal dental culture, the patchwork dentistry, and the health care culture that said it was okay for people to needlessly lose teeth to disease and ignorance. But it went beyond that; after a serious accident and going through the process of regaining her health, she decided to transform her dental practice from one aimed at treating as many patients as possible into a practice aimed at treating as many of the needs of her patients as possible.

Why does she serve the clients she serves? To bring dental health services to the community they live in. She also wants to provide these services in a calm, serene environment that helps reduce stress and anxiety. Bringing all the treatment options under one roof so her patients don't have the stress of looking for the right specialist for their dental needs is one way to do that. Another is to combine comfort and technology to create fantastic smiles while treating every patient in a warm, caring manner as if they were a guest in her home. Finally, she's also focused on providing the critical education patients need to end the problem of poor dental health that comes from ignorance, while also creating personalized plans to move people toward a level of dental care that's second to none.

The Solution

After we understood the why behind Dr. Rementer's practice and the challenges she was facing, we presented a more comprehensive solution to fulfill the practice's needs. We determined the practice needed a logo structure that unified the organization across all its locations while having an element of differentiation to provide quick identification for each. This new system would extend beyond a simple logo and identity system to become the foundation for a new comprehensive brand and brand strategy embodying the mission Dr. Rementer set forth during her recovery.

We understood Dr. Rementer would be better served with a comprehensive package with a more robust branding and identity system. This determination allowed us to move forward with foundational research and strategy development.

What Research and Strategy Development has to do with Branding

When dealing with branding and strategy, you must come from a place of education and understanding. We obtain a great deal by speaking with clients and pulling out information about their practice, personality, vision for the future, and what issues they see as challenging. However, if we stop there, we are performing a disservice to our clients. We could provide them with something they would probably be happy with, which may even solve their perceived problem, but are we solving the issue or just applying a patch?

For these reasons, branding is not a done-for-you service but a done-with-you service. Anyone who tells you they will produce your branding without interaction is NOT providing you with a comprehensive and customized brand solution.

The Research Required for Branding and Brand Strategy Development

Depending on the client's need, budget and comprehensiveness of the project, the following studies, analyses, audits, and determinations will be made: *(Please note this is not a comprehensive list.)* Competitive Analysis, Customer Analysis, Positioning Strategy, Differentiator Exploration, SWOT Analysis, Patient/Target Audience, Social Media Analysis, Internal Client Audit, Gaps & Ideas Study, Archetypes, Visual Personas, Brand Voice, Tone & Vocabulary, Positioning Strategy, Core Message, Brand

Story, Audience Journey, Buyers Journey, Keywords, Color, Touchpoint Audit.

You may notice an overlap in some of the research your business coach, marketing team, and brand strategist are performing. Each is looking for something slightly different in the research. Still, you can assist all parties working with you to grow your practice by sharing the resulting reports and strategy documents. Sharing research may not eliminate an individual service provider's need for doing their own research and development, but it can assist them in knowing what strategies they are already working with or have tried in the past. This allows them to develop a more comprehensive plan to move the needle in a positive direction.

Essentially, a brand strategy document serves as a comprehensive guide, ensuring all branding efforts align with the brand's core values, goals and vision. It is both a strategic tool and a reference document that ensures the brand remains consistent and true to its identity across all communications and interactions.

A brand strategy document is one of the main deliverables you receive when you work with a brand strategist. This document serves as a comprehensive guide that ensures all efforts by the branding agency align with the practice's approved core values, goals and vision This document should be used daily and referenced by your employees and marketing team when they are engaged in any activity that needs to be "on brand."

The components that are typically included in a Brand Strategy document include:

Brand Overview: The brand overview contains the practice's fundamental principles. These include its mission, which we define as the business's core purpose. The mission also answers the question of its primary goals and objectives. Next, we delve into the practice's vision for the future. The practice vision should paint a picture in response to the following: Where does the company see itself in the future? What is the long-term aim? The final piece of this section deals with your practice values. These principles and beliefs guide the practice's actions and decisions.

Competitive Analysis: The competitive analysis examines the market landscape by taking an overview of the industry and the key players in your location. This is facilitated through the completion of a Strengths, Weaknesses, Opportunities and Threats (SWOT) analysis of each competitor's brand in its current position. Analysis is also taken of their social media, marketing materials, and other touchpoints.

Target Audience: When developing the target audience, it's tempting to say "everyone," but everyone means you're focused on no one. User personas (or avatars) will be developed for each type of patient you have. These fictional patients are more than just a set of demographics (age, gender, location, income, and other measurable statistics). They need to have a complete psychographic build-out as well; this includes their values, beliefs, interests, lifestyles, and other qualitative attributes. Only by creating a complete "person" can your avatar provide insights into who you are trying to reach, where you can find them, and how to connect with them.

Brand Positioning: So many marketing and business professionals tell you about the importance of your unique value proposition (UVP). They are right. You need something that is going to set your practice apart from competitors. But it's not limited to only your UVP. When examining your brand positioning and developing your positioning statement (a concise description of the brand's unique value and target audience), we expand the elements of setting your practice apart into areas not typically considered by business and marketing coaches. Brand positioning explores what differentiates your practice, which can be achieved an unlimited number of ways. Through identification, presentation and amplification, your practice can carve out a niche and raise your practice above the noise of "others" in your industry. When you become ***"The Dentist"*** you no longer compete with dentists. You have become the only dentist for implants, cosmetics, seniors, special-need individuals, podcasters, hockey players, golfers, CEOs, etc. The list is endless.

The Tone of Voice: When we discuss tone of voice, most people assume we're just talking about writing. However, tone of voice is about more than that; it's about the way your practice communicates. It's the personality it expresses in its writing, speaking and videos. How does the brand communicate its messages across various channels? Is the brand formal, playful, serious, or empathetic?

Visual Identity: Branding visual identity covers the development and application of the practice logo, color palette, typography, photos, illustrations, and other visual media. These are established through the design process, and usage standards and guidelines are established and preserved in a Style Guide.

Visual identity is not limited to printed and digital applications. Your brand's visual identity needs to be considered across all elements of your practice. This can include everything from paint colors to fabric selections, uniform colors, signage, artwork, and video displays.

Brand Messaging: What message are you trying to convey across your brand? This should be driven by the core elements of your brand (values, purpose, mission) and reflected in the short, catchy phrases that encapsulate the brand's essence, such as your tagline, slogan and core statements.

Your brand story conveys the brand's history in a narrative interwoven with its core elements and provides an engaging/inspiring way of connecting your target audience with the brand, which can help produce an emotional connection. Brand stories can be used to develop a sense of commonality with your desired audience/patients by exposing a pain point, showing a solution is possible, and describing the path to get there.

Brand Touchpoints: Touchpoints cover *ALL* ways your practice interacts with potential patients, existing patients, staff, and the general public. A short list includes physical touchpoints, such as storefronts, packaging, business cards, etc.; digital touchpoints, such as websites, social media profiles, email campaigns, etc.; and human touchpoints, such as customer service interactions and sales processes.

Goals and KPIs: Often, goals and Key Performance Indicators (KPIs) are not included or considered when dentists develop their branding, but branding must have goals attached. These goals can be quantifiable, allowing you to develop a brand strategy that is measurable and provides you with the metrics you need to understand the return on investment (ROI) of your branding efforts.

It's important to develop both short-term and long-term goals. Your short-term goals should consist of the milestones you want to achieve in the upcoming months, while your long-term goals should focus on what you want to achieve in the coming years.

Relate every goal to a KPI. The KPI provides the metrics you will use to measure the success of the brand strategy.

Implementation and Guidelines: These are the physical "deliverables" of a branding project. The *Brand Guidelines* or *Brand Style Guide* details how brand elements should be applied in different situations. This includes components such as the logo, colors, typography, iconography, stationary, signage, graphic elements, video standards, presentation templates, etc. The *Content Strategy* is the plan for content creation and distribution. This contains elements such as the tone of voice, text formatting and heading hierarchy, storyboarding, and channels for distribution. The *Engagement Strategy* is a document that details how the brand will interact with its audience. These can each be provided individually or as a section of the final brand strategy document.

The Implementation

In developing a logo mark that would most accurately represent the organization while maintaining visual cues as to the individual offices, we first explored the character of the practice and its founder, Dr. Rementer.

After making a discovery, we recognized Dr. Rementer loved the ocean and desired to bring the calm and serenity she found there into her practice. She also wanted a mark that could speak to her desire to be an all-encompassing dental service, eliminating the need for her patients to seek care outside of the practice for specialty services.

The mark we developed answered these needs as it could be perceived as a smile, a wave, and a roof under which all her services could be housed. By shifting the color of the mark and replacing the overarching location name (North Carolina) with the individual practice location, we were able to provide her with a mark that could grow with her practice while allowing both staff and patients a quick point of reference to ensure they were in the correct office location.

We also identified imagery and colors that reinforce the calming nature of the ocean theme, which was used as the identifying colors for each of the practice offices, as well as a secondary palette that would be integrated across all offices.

MEASURING YOUR BRANDING ROI

Effective branding is often overlooked in health care, where exceptional patient care is the primary focus. However, a robust branding strategy is essential for attracting new patients in today's competitive landscape. While branding is often seen as an abstract concept, adopting an ROI-focused approach can provide concrete, measurable results. This comprehensive guide is designed to help health care providers understand the benefits of an ROI-focused branding strategy and how to implement it effectively.

Understanding ROI in branding is crucial as it refers to the returns you get from your branding investments. These can be measured in various ways, such as increased patient engagement, higher patient retention rates, or even direct financial gains. Health care providers need to ensure their branding efforts are cost-effective and yield tangible results.

The first step in any ROI-focused approach is to align your branding efforts with your business goals. Whether you aim to increase patient retention, attract a new demographic, or expand your services, your branding should serve these objectives. Define your goals clearly and tailor your strategy to meet these objectives. For example, suppose your goal is to attract younger patients. In that case, your marketing might focus on digital platforms and use a more modern esthetic or terminology that aligns more closely with this demographic.

Next, set up KPIs to measure the effectiveness of your branding efforts. These should be aligned with your business goals and provide actionable insights. Choose KPIs that are directly related to your business goals and use analytics tools to track them, ensuring you set up proper tracking mechanisms to collect accurate data.

Effective budget management is crucial for calculating ROI. Knowing where your money goes can help you assess the most cost-effective branding activities. Allocate your overall branding budget into different categories like digital advertising, print materials, and staff training to help track spending more effectively.

With your KPIs and budget in place, you're ready to roll out your branding strategies. These could range from a new logo and website redesign to social media campaigns and patient outreach programs. Implement your planned branding activities and monitor their performance using the tracking codes, analytics tools, and KPIs you've set up. This will not only help you measure ROI but also make real-time adjustments to your strategies.

Data collection and analysis play a pivotal role in any ROI-focused approach. They provide the insights needed to assess the effectiveness of your branding efforts. Once the data is collected, it's crucial to analyze it to understand what's working and what's not. Look for patterns or trends that could provide actionable insights. This step is key to making informed decisions and optimizing your branding strategies for maximum impact and returns.

The final step in an ROI-focused approach is to make informed decisions based on your data analysis. During this step, you'll see the value of focusing on ROI. Identify which branding activities yield the best ROI and continue or even scale up these strategies. If certain activities are not providing a good ROI, it may be time to adjust or eliminate them.

Adopting an ROI-focused approach to branding allows health care providers to quantify the success of their branding efforts. By setting clear goals, tracking KPIs, and making data-driven decisions, health care providers can optimize their branding strategies for maximum impact and returns. It's important to remember branding is not a one-time activity but an ongoing process. Regularly review your KPIs and iterate and optimize your branding efforts. Consulting branding experts or agencies can provide valuable insights and specialized guidance to help you stay on top of your branding game.

Branding is essential to any health care practice but shouldn't drain resources with no measurable returns. An ROI-focused approach ensures every dollar spent on branding is an investment in your practice's growth and success.

Guest Chapter by Dan S. Kennedy

"I Didn't Sign Up For THIS"

You went to dental school, you did *not* major in advertising and marketing. You aspire to excellence with your clinical skills and with patient care. You *haven't* been thinking about having the best Invisalign® or implant or other dental advertising in your area. You certainly *didn't* plan on managing print, direct-mail, multiple websites and "funnels," a dozen different social media channels, YouTube and TikTok video production, constant demand for new content, possibly radio, even TV. Add to that the need for comprehensive follow-up on calls or site visits with no appointment, missed appointments, and appointments that didn't result in a sale. How about data mining from your own patient base as it grows for specific, high probability targets for outreach about specific treatments or services? Being a direct-response copywriter capable of producing results in an attention competitive environment?

I've worked directly with dentists since 1981, and with groups of them through and in collaboration with a long list of top practice consultants and coaches, including Jay Geier/Scheduling Institute, Linda Miles, Dr. Tom Orent, Greg Stanley/Whitehall, and others. My current private clients in the profession include NUVIA, a fast growing national chain of implant clinics, at 36 and counting; a wonderful dentist and his wife, Dr. Len and Nancy Anglis, with a very upscale, thriving practice; and Dr. Emily Letran, with a great practice and a coaching program for dentists. My clientele has always been and continues to be diverse, as I have worked across more than 100 product and service categories in 50 years. But I've been breaking the news, telling the often very unwelcome facts of life to dentists a lot for a lot of years, as they plaintively cry, "But I didn't sign up for *that!*"

You may *not* know what you signed up for in private practice, but here are the "harsh realities":

1: **Your deliverables are <u>not</u> your business**. Dentistry; patient treatment and care; a well managed office with friendly staff, these are (just) deliverables. They are (just) the ante to get a seat at the business table. Nothing less but nothing more. *Then* the game begins.

2: **The "best" dentist in town is rarely the most successful, in business and financial terms.** More often than not, the "best" dentists aren't even in the top 10 practices, and those "best" dentists are frustrated by it, indignant about it, mystified by it. They have, by some, been taught and they have developed a near religious belief that excellence in dentistry entitles them to excellent practice growth, stability, income and produced wealth. This is a fantastical belief about how things SHOULD work, but it is willful blindness to how things DO work. You must jettison *any* "entitlement attitude." If you expect to do very well purely because you are an excellent dentist, you expect way too much. In business, we all get what we intentionally, proactively attract and interest and persuade, *not* what we think we deserve.

3: **You are in the direct marketing business**. The best way to gain a quick but thorough understanding of this "strange" fact and to know what to do about it is my book, *NO B.S. GUIDE TO DIRECT MARKETING FOR NON-DIRECT MARKETING BUSINESSES, 4TH EDITION*. Your actual business is marketing, your deliverables are dentistry. Unless and until you embrace *this* reality and develop knowledge and interest in your real business and enthusiasm for it, you will struggle for growth and for profitability, and suffer growing frustration with practice over time. When you *do* embrace *this*, dramatic, fast quantum leaps in success are possible.

Broadly speaking, there is an income and wealth pyramid in dentistry. It has 1% at its peak, the doctors taking home 7-figures and wisely investing to grow personal wealth. Four percent doing very well in business and financial terms. Another 15% in the low to mid 6-figure bracket, for income extracted from practice. All together, a top 20%. The bigger, wider, fatter bottom of the pyramid divides 40% making (only) a decent living and 40% barely meeting payroll and paying bills but never getting ahead at all. The difference between the 80% and the 20% is not at all what you might think or what you might hope. It is that the further up this pyramid you look, the more you find "marketers of" dentistry. The lower you go on the pyramid, the more you find "doers of" dentistry. The bottom 40% is comprised of factory workers in white coats. They come every morning when the whistle blows, lunch pail in hand, check in at the front desk, and disappear into "the back" to "do teeth." The staff runs the practice and runs them. They *don't like* marketing and want as little to do with it as possible. Toward the top of the pyramid you find dentists who are advertising, marketing and business enthusiasts. They've learned to like their real business. Many I've worked with or closely observed did not like it at first but made the mindset adjustments required for the success they wanted. Maturity, after all, is much about not letting your likes and dislikes hurt you. And just for the record, there is no marketer-gene you were born without. My speaking colleague on tour for 9 years, the great Zig Ziglar, said he checked the newspaper birth announcements every day of his life and saw little baby boys born and little baby girls, but never once a little baby salesman. It's an acquired taste, acquired fascination, acquired skill.

By the way, marketing is fun. Developing wildly successful marketing for your practice can be the most fun you ever have with your clothes on.

4: **You dare not simply abdicate it.** You will be bombarded by "agencies" and a myriad of other vendors who promise to take these marketing responsibilities entirely off your hands. If you inherited way too much money, this is a great way to get rid of some, if flying to Vegas is too time-consuming. You CAN delegate a lot, but you need to understand what you are delegating, and collaborate and oversee and at times direct.

This is where, for example, my friend and client Parthiv Shah comes in, with his Dental Growth Machine® and his Sell More Implants® system and services. He has brilliantly taken my most potent strategies and mined other sources to "systemize" both internal and external marketing for dental practices. He can document considerable success. He is also a great data scientist, adept at avatar patient matching. He even, very unusually, holds U.S. Patents on marketing processes. But, but, but, I would still never recommend "Do it for me, Parthiv, while I play dentist or play golf," any more than I would suggest you just write a check to a contractor to build you a million dollar custom home without you seeing and having input into the design plans.

I invited Parthiv to be the lead co-author with me on the NO B.S. GUIDE TO SUCCESSFUL MARKETING AUTOMATION AND A.I., and un-humbly recommend it as a great overview of how your marketing can be automated for you. Much of what I rattled off at the start of this chapter *can* be. Because you are and want to be a dentist, you have no choice but to delegate—or stagnate. The trick is to delegate knowledgeably. Incidentally, about likes and dislikes, I probably dislike "tech" more than you dislike marketing. I use almost none of it personally, and I'd rather have a root canal without a topical done by a drunk dentist than go online, let alone to Facebook. But tech has revolutionized direct marketing, so I have not let my likes and dislikes hurt me. I'm very knowledgeable and I constantly create winning advertising for social media, successful scripts for webcasts, and full no-fail follow-up systems integrating email, text, etc. with good old-fashioned mail. I can delegate what I don't want to *do* only by knowing what I want *done*.

Please, Don't Be Amish

In every profession, dentistry included, at least the bottom 80% act as if Amish. They get into a circle looking inward at each other. Newcomers conform, to fit in, mostly without ever questioning what they see and copycat or what they are told by "the elders." It is intellectually incestuous. As with actual incest, those participating are stunted and even get dumber and dumber. Innovation is two mules to one plow instead of one. Marketing incest is the worst aspect, because almost all great breakthroughs in dental marketing have come and will come from outside the community, not bubbling up from inside it. Your success requires an open, curious, observant mind.

Actually, the Amish are great entrepreneurs and great marketers, using both offline and online media. They discovered a few decades back that just crafting the very best furniture in the world or doing the finest kitchen remodels or roof replacement or having wonderful farm-to-table restaurants was not nearly enough to meet their business and financial needs and ambitions. I live near Amish communities and, because I own Standardbred racehorses, have gotten to know many. I've learned how they changed their attitudes about entitlement and became smart about advertising, marketing, multi-channel distribution. So, in this respect, go ahead and be Amish! Just don't be "old" Amish, engaged in closed circle imitation and small boxed-in thinking.

#

DAN S. KENNEDY is a much sought after direct marketing strategy consultant and copywriter, helping build brands and businesses like Perfect Smile® and Proactiv®, America's #1 acne treatment, MiracleEar®, and Medicare Express®. He is the author of the bestselling series of "NO B.S." books, including the most recent *No B.S. Guide to Succeeding In Business by Breaking ALL The Rules*. As a speaker, his long career includes 9 years on the largest public seminar tour in America, alongside four former U.S. Presidents, countless Hollywood and sports celebrities, great marketing founder-CEOs like Debbi Fields (Mrs. Fields Cookies) and Jim McCann (1-800-Flowers), and legendary speakers including Zig Ziglar, Brian Tracy, Jim Rohn and Tom Hopkins. His own seminar events have featured celebrity-entrepreneurs like Gene Simmons (KISS), Joan Rivers, George Foreman and Kathy Ireland The entrepreneurs' organization he founded can be looked in on at MagneticMarketing.com. Over 30,000 dentists, chiropractors and other health care professionals have been in his audiences.

Afterword
Dental Marketing Breakthrough

After reading this book, you might feel like your mind is racing with ideas. What should you focus on first? How should you begin? Don't worry—this chapter is here to guide you.

The entire purpose of this book is to show that you, as a dentist, have the ability to grow your practice by selling more implants. But beyond that, it's about something far greater—it's about changing lives in ways that ripple far beyond the dental chair.

When you help patients reclaim their smile with implants, yes, you're restoring their teeth, but as importantly, you're restoring their ability to enjoy the simple pleasures that make life worth living.

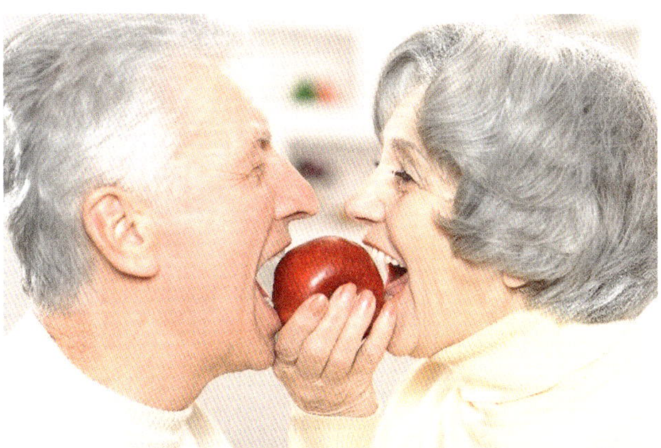

Think about the joy on someone's face as they take a confident bite into a crisp apple for the first time in years or the satisfaction they feel savoring their favorite steak without hesitation. These are life-affirming milestones for someone who thought they'd never experience them again.

But it's not just about food. Dental implants restore dignity and confidence. Patients who once avoided family photos because of embarrassment flash radiant smiles in every picture.

People who avoided speaking up in meetings or social situations, afraid their missing or loose teeth would draw unwanted attention, stand tall, and express themselves without fear. The transformation is profound—it's physical, emotional and even social.

As a dentist, you can give people a piece of their life back. You're helping someone rediscover the confidence to go on dates, to laugh out loud, to reconnect with old friends, and to show up fully in their lives. You're not just fixing teeth; you're giving people the tools to live without limits.

By providing implants, you're giving your patients the ability to step into the world with renewed self-esteem and the assurance that they deserve to be seen, heard and valued.

When you choose to focus on this part of your practice, you're not just growing your business; you're becoming a catalyst for life-changing transformations. That's a powerful and deeply rewarding mission, and it's why the work you do matters so much.

Let me tell you about a moment that brought this realization into sharp focus for me.

In December 2024, I was on a plane to Los Angeles, laptop open, working on an event landing page for a dental summit. Sitting next to me was an elderly woman who had been quietly observing. Finally, with a polite curiosity, she asked, "Are you a dentist? Do you do implants?"

I smiled and shook my head. "No, I'm not a dentist. But I help dentists sell more implants and build systems to help them do it better."

Her face lit up as she leaned closer, revealing a radiant smile. "Well, I have a full arch," she said proudly. "And I love them. They feel so natural, and I love how they look."

She wasn't exaggerating. Her smile was incredible—bright, even and full of life. I couldn't resist asking who her dentist was, and when she mentioned his name, I realized he was someone I had worked with in Irvine, California. It felt like a full-circle moment.

We continued talking, and I learned her name was Grace. At 88 years old, she had the energy and spirit of someone much younger. We chatted about her life and my father, who is 89. Sadly, my dad doesn't have enough bone in his jaw for implants and has to rely on dentures. Seeing Grace's vibrant smile, I couldn't help but think about how transformative implants can be—not just for appearance but for confidence and quality of life.

Then, in a moment of conspiratorial charm, Grace leaned in closer, lowering her voice as if sharing a secret. "You know, I don't tell my friends this," she began with a playful twinkle in her eye, "but I love how easy it is to care for my teeth. Just a toothbrush and a water-pick every day. That's it!"

She grinned, her voice bubbling with delight. "None of that popping them in a cup with those fizzy cleaning tablets like my friends must do. I'll tell you, I'm so glad I don't have to deal with that!"

Her joy was infectious, and I found myself laughing along with her. Grace was proud, and rightfully so. Her implants had given her a freedom and ease that made her truly happy.

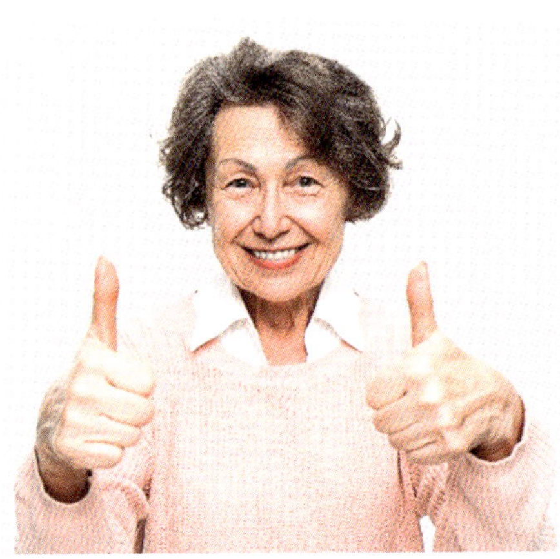

As we said our goodbyes, she looked at me with sincerity. "Thank you," she said softly. "You're doing good work. You're in the right business."

Moments like that are a reminder of why we do what we do. This book isn't about making money—neither for me through its sales nor for you through selling more implants. It's about educating patients.

It's about offering solutions when natural teeth are no longer an option—implants, full arches, cosmetic treatments, and sedation dentistry that make people feel vibrant again.

Implants may not add years to our lives, but they absolutely add life to our years. And that's something worth smiling about.

It's with patients like Grace in mind that I developed the **Dental Marketing Breakthrough**—a starting point designed to help you connect with and educate your patients.

If you're looking for where to begin, I suggest starting here. This is a small taste of the full power of the **Dental Growth Machine**, but make no mistake—it's incredibly effective.

Here's what it includes:

- **Two Simple Funnels**
- **One Small Marketing Automation**
- **8–10 Patient Education and Case Presentation Assets**, all focused on helping patients like Grace.

The Purpose?

To educate your patients, plain and simple. Patients like Grace need to understand their situation before they'll say yes to treatment. Why? Because many patients will say no—not because they don't need the treatment, but because they don't trust you yet. They're afraid. Afraid of the commitment, afraid of the cost, and, frankly, afraid of you.

Your job isn't just to diagnose and recommend treatment, but to calm their fears. Help them understand their current situation, their treatment options, and—most importantly—the **real cost of doing nothing**. You've got to answer the questions they're too embarrassed or overwhelmed to ask.

And here's the truth you know they don't yet realize: Once the bone is gone, it's gone. God gave us a small window of opportunity to replace the teeth Mother Nature took away. If you don't act, that window slams shut forever. And when the bone is gone, your options become severely limited. Like my father, who waited too long, patients may be left with no choice but to wear dentures—a far less comfortable, less functional, and less satisfying solution—all because they didn't act in time.

Your role isn't to "sell more implants." Your role is to **educate and act before it's too late.** The **Dental Marketing Breakthrough** helps you do that.

When you educate your patients thoroughly, build trust and calm their fears, the natural byproduct is more implant cases. And that growth is what justifies the nontrivial investment in bringing home, installing, and customizing the full **Dental Growth Machine**.

The **Dental Marketing Breakthrough**, as described in this chapter, is a miniature, minimum-viable version of **Dental Growth Machine**. It's the fastest, simplest way to begin transforming the way you educate your patients and grow your practice.

Start here and you'll help patients like Grace and set your practice on a path toward significant, sustainable growth.

When dentists partner with me and invest in the **Dental Growth Machine**, the **Dental Marketing Breakthrough** serves as the initial step. Over the first 90 days, for a modest investment, we install, customize and deploy these assets to determine if proceeding with the full system aligns with your practice's goals.

Most dentists love the results and choose to move forward with the Dental Growth Machine, and this is where the real transformation begins.

The **Dental Growth Machine** includes:

ADVANCED PATIENT EDUCATION MATERIALS

- **Smile Book**: A picture is worth a thousand words. This book acts as a visual showcase of your success stories, highlighting the transformations of your patients. Prospects see the joy and confidence your work brings, and they are inspired to become the next success story in your book.
- **Case Presentation Package**: A tailored set of tools that helps your team address objections and deliver persuasive presentations. It includes personalized letters, step-by-step guides, and service booklets designed to handle objections, build trust, and guide prospects toward saying YES.
- **Implant Pricing Guide**: A transparent breakdown of costs associated with dental implants, including financing options. This builds trust and helps patients feel like they are making informed decisions about their oral health investments.
- **Educational Reports**: "Choosing the Right Dentist" and "The Implant Report," each with dedicated landing pages and follow-up emails. These resources address patients' concerns, positioning your practice as the authoritative choice and guiding them toward committing to implants.
- **Influence and Persuasion Aids**: A series of single-page client nurture and prospect conversion aids, drawing on the influence and persuasion principles of Dr. Christopher Phelps and Dr. Robert Cialdini. Using tools like reciprocity, social proof, and authority, we help answer common questions and ease worries clients might have. This makes it easier for them to say yes.
- **Automated Follow-Up Systems**: Streamlined processes that maintain consistent and personalized communication with patients, making them feel valued and informed throughout their journey.
- **Comprehensive Marketing Campaigns**: Targeted strategies that effectively attract and retain patients, expanding your practice's reach and impact.
- **Data-Driven Analytics**: Tools to monitor and assess the performance of marketing efforts, providing insights that drive continuous improvement and success.

As a dentist, your mission extends beyond the dental chair. It's about transforming lives—enabling patients to enjoy their favorite foods, smile confidently, and maintain their dignity as they age. Our **Dental Growth Machine** is designed to support this mission by providing tools and strategies that take your practice to the next level and help you connect with your prospects and better serve your patients.

While the **Dental Marketing Breakthrough** offers a solid foundation, the full **Dental Growth Machine** delves deeper, equipping you with advanced resources to effectively educate and engage your patients.

The insights you've learned in this book are actionable; you can implement it all independently, collaborate with a vendor of your choice, or partner with us at eLaunchers to experience firsthand why hundreds of dentists trust us to grow their practices. For more details on each asset mentioned and to access ready-to-use samples and swipe files, please visit https://swipefilesandsamples.com.

My mission isn't about my personal financial gain. It's about making a meaningful impact—helping patients like Grace and supporting the dentists dedicated to their care. We want to empower men and women to smile confidently and maintain their oral health well into their later years. As my friend and client, Dr. Omar, aptly states, "Patients should pass away with their teeth in their mouth, not in a cup." This philosophy embodies the essence of the **Dental Marketing Breakthrough**.

As you finish this chapter, take a moment to think about the incredible difference you can make as a dentist focused on implants. Every smile you help restore gives your patients back their confidence and improves their lives.

Remember Grace's story and all the others who've found joy and dignity through your work. Let their experiences inspire you to see your practice not just as a business but as a mission to make a real difference. Use the tips and tools in this chapter to support this important work.

Starting today, focus on educating your patients with care and clarity. Build trust by addressing their fears and questions, and you'll see your practice grow both in numbers and in the hearts of your community. Your dedication and genuine care will set you apart, creating lasting relationships and a thriving practice.

You have the power to truly change lives, helping people smile confidently and live without limits. Here's to your success and the many lives you'll touch along the way.

Glossary

$(COH \geq COB)^t$: The contribution of overhead (COH) always must be greater than the cost of breathing. This is a big point of contention with many people I talk to. When they are out of compliance, they call it an "investment." I say, "But you are losing money," and they say, "If you look at it that way, my business will never grow!"

Case presentation: A print asset that helps convert any team member into an effective salesperson.

COB: The out-of-pocket expenses at zero revenue, also known as the cost of breathing.

Important note. Revenue increases when the costs of transactions decrease (or remain low), and the number of transactions increases. To maintain or increase profitability, entrepreneurs need to keep COS, COGS, and COB down.

COGS: The cost of goods (or services) sold.

Competitive analysis: Take a hard look at your competitive position in your market and find out who is doing what to whom.

COS: The cost of acquiring the sale (commissions, marketing expenses, etc.).

CVP analysis: The cost-volume-profit analysis is used to determine what you can cheerfully afford to spend to acquire a new client.

Dental Data Protocol: This is about helping you find and collect ideal patients in your own database who have a desperate need for dental implants and the ability to say yes to treatment you recommend.

Geofencing: Setting up a virtual perimeter around your location.

Marketing automation plan: A way to design a perfect customer life cycle process and set of interlinking, technology-enabled systems that facilitate business growth and profitability.

Pixel estate: Your website and online presence where your prospects and patients engage with you.

PRISM research: This gives you an unprecedented advantage in the marketplace and allows you to reach out across your community and identify the ideal people who can benefit from a product or service you offer.

Shock and awe: An effective asset that engages your prospects, excites them, and helps convert them into patients.

SWOT analysis: Use this method to identify and analyze your and your practice's strengths, weaknesses, opportunities and threats.

The TRIAD KLT: People buy from people they know, like and trust (KLT). The goal of a persuasive marketing campaign is to establish the TRIAD KLT.

Appendix 1
Resources

Today, I continue to help business owners achieve their next level of success. Whether it's setting up a funnel that results in a million dollars in sales or redesigning a website to attract more customers, my clients love the documented revenue growth they experience in their business after hiring me.

And this makes me happy. Helping businesses grow is my purpose and passion; with this in mind, I am offering you the following gifts.

First, I'm giving you access to my bookshelf, freemarketingbooks.com. Here, you will find several books I've written and co-written on various business growth-related topics. These resources are full of valuable information and actionable strategies you can apply in your business today to move the profit needle higher.

Second, I'm giving you access to my Business Growth System, freegrowthsystem.com. Here, you will discover how to add $100K to your revenue within one year. You will have access to powerful marketing assets you can start using immediately. We use the same marketing assets to generate millions of dollars in revenue for our business and professional practice clients year after year.

I hope you take me up on these offers; you will be glad you did.

Generally, I am extremely busy helping my clients achieve their business growth goals. Still, I will always make time to answer your questions and help in every way I can. If you are interested in taking your business to a new level, then please send me a text or give me a call at 301-873-5791. Together, we can take the next step to maximize your revenue while minimizing costs and growing your business with speed and predictability.

Thank you. I look forward to hearing from you soon.

Sincerely,

Parthiv Shah

ADDITIONAL RESOURCES

Some of the technologies I use and recommend:

- Marketing automation: Keap, ClickFunnels, HubSpot, ActiveCampaign, GoHighLevel, Thryv
- Graphic design: Adobe InDesign, Illustrator, Photoshop, Apple Pages, Microsoft Publisher, Canva
- Web hosting: wpengine.com
- Website design: Wordpress, Click Funnels or HubSpot CMS
- Landing pages: HubSpot, Clickfunnels.com, Keap
- Membership sites: CustomerHub, imember360, WordPress Wishlist, Memberium
- Dashboard and Data Visualization: HubSpot Databox, Google Data Studio, Microsoft Power BI
- Social media integration with HubSpot
- Application integration with Zapier
- PCI compliance and e-commerce credit card processing: Authorize.net and QuickBooks Online
- Video editing: Adobe Premiere Pro, Final Cut Pro, VideoScribe
- Cloud computing: Microsoft Office 365, Google Workspace

- Online calendar and appointment scheduling: HubSpot, Keap, Thryv, ClickFunnels
- Note-taking: Microsoft OneNote
- Mobile technology for the road: Samsung Phone with Pen, and Microsoft Surface Pro
- Cloud file storage: Dropbox, Box, Microsoft OneDrive, Google Drive
- Project management and team collaboration: Monday.com
- Email marketing (small budget or free tools): Go High Level
- Video recording and editing training: There are plenty of free training videos available on YouTube. My favorite video editing courses are from Samsung and DJI. I absolutely love my DJI Osmo Pocket 3 video camera and its companion app
- Copywriting: Montblanc and Cartier
- Text messaging: Simple Texting, Keap, Thryv
- Call capture and reverse data append: Ring Central, MVP Call ProList research: srds.com and acculeads.com
- Data intelligence and data cleansing: Validity Brite-verify and Validity Everest
- Online data storage: MySQL, MS SQL, Microsoft Sharepoint
- Preferred programming language: PHP
- Online meeting: Zoom
- Artificial Intelligence: Tools too many to mention and this is a moving landscape. Visit www.elaunchers.com/tech-updates for a complete line up

Appendix 2
Samples and Swipe Files

OK, folks, as promised, this is the chapter I give you access to samples of sales funnels, e-newsletters, shock and awe packages, case presentation packages, long-term nurture packages, and much more.

I have used each of these assets with my dental clients to help them grow their practices, reach and connect with more qualified leads, and send their profits soaring to new heights they never dreamed possible.

> *"Parthiv is brilliant at integrating publicity, marketing and sales into both online and offline deliveries coordinated for maximum impact. His concepts of marketing automation help deliver more new clients and more dollars where it counts the most, your wallet."*
>
> - Dr. Charles W. Martin

This chapter goes into great detail. If you are reading this online, there will be links you can follow, but if you have a hard copy in hand right now, please visit https://swipefilesandsamples.com for a more in-depth look at all you're about to see.

Please remember, these are examples you can use for guidance, a jumping-off point to start your creative process. Still, we have created these copyrighted materials specifically using bespoke copy for our clients. These are not shared with the intent that you will take and use them verbatim.

With that said, let's begin.

IMPLANT SALES FUNNELS

You now know all about how effective sales funnels can be in helping you attract the attention of your ideal prospects and converting them into satisfied patients who eagerly refer everyone they know to your practice.

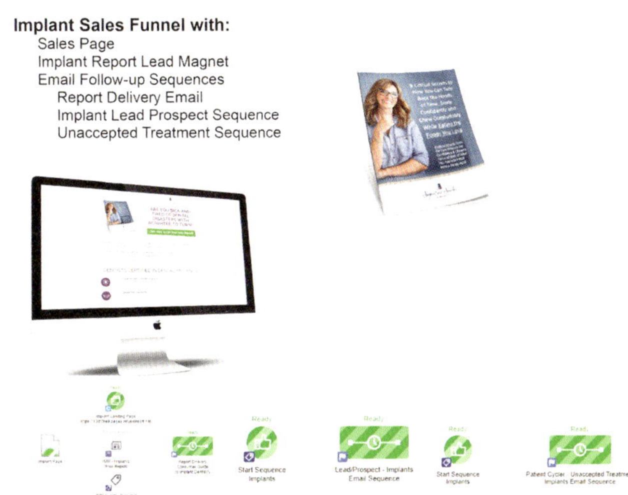

An implant sales funnel consists of several parts:

- The sales page or landing page: An effective sales or landing page will capture your prospect's attention with a good headline, "**Are You Tired of HATING The Way Your Teeth Look When You Smile and Wish You Could Speak and Laugh with Confidence and Ease**?" It will then tease what they can learn if they download a special report.

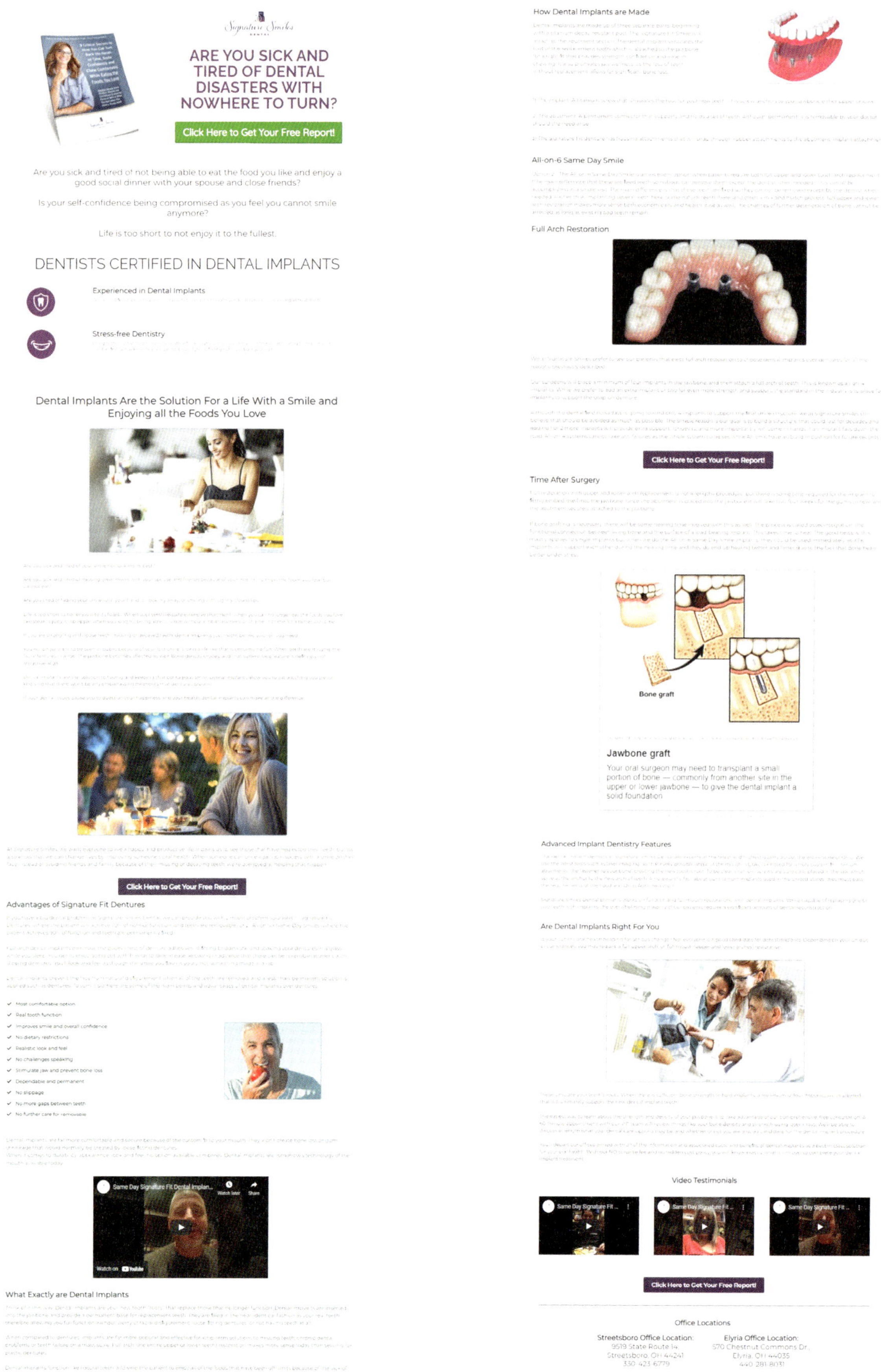
ARE YOU SICK AND TIRED OF DENTAL DISASTERS WITH NOWHERE TO TURN?
Click Here to Get Your Free Report!
Are you sick and tired of not being able to eat the food you like and enjoy a good social dinner with your spouse and close friends?
Is your self-confidence being compromised as you feel you cannot smile anymore?
Life is too short to not enjoy it to the fullest.
DENTISTS CERTIFIED IN DENTAL IMPLANTS
Experienced in Dental Implants
Stress-free Dentistry
Dental Implants Are the Solution For a Life With a Smile and Enjoying all the Foods You Love
Click Here to Get Your Free Report!
Advantages of Signature Fit Dentures
Most comfortable option
Real tooth function
Improves smile and overall confidence
No dietary restrictions
Realistic look and feel
No challenges speaking
Stimulate jaw and prevent bone loss
Dependable and permanent
No slippage
No more gaps between teeth
No further care for removable
What Exactly are Dental Implants
How Dental Implants are Made
All-on-6 Same Day Smile
Full Arch Restoration
Click Here to Get Your Free Report!
Time After Surgery
Bone graft
Jawbone graft
Your oral surgeon may need to transplant a small portion of bone — commonly from another site in the upper or lower jawbone — to give the dental implant a solid foundation.
Advanced Implant Dentistry Features
Are Dental Implants Right For You
Video Testimonials
Click Here to Get Your Free Report!
Office Locations
Streetsboro Office Location:
9519 State Route 14,
Streetsboro, OH 44241
330-423-6779
Elyria Office Location:
570 Chestnut Commons Dr.,
Elyria, OH 44035
440-281-8031

- The implant report lead magnet: To receive the report, prospects must provide their name, phone number and email address. If they'd like a physical copy of the report delivered to their doorway, they must also provide their mailing address. The report is a powerful piece that will answer their questions, address their fears, concerns, and objections, and single them out as ideal candidates for dental implant treatment. If qualified prospects read this report all the way through, chances are high they will reach out to you, ready to say yes to dental implants.
- Email follow-up sequences: Once you have their contact information, prospects receive a series of emails meant to educate them and entice them to contact your office, ready to accept the treatment you recommend. These emails include:
  1. Report delivery email
  2. Implant lead prospect sequence
  3. Unaccepted treatment sequence

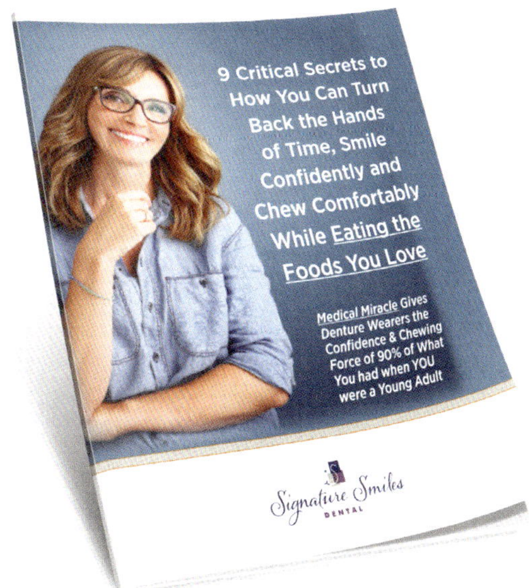

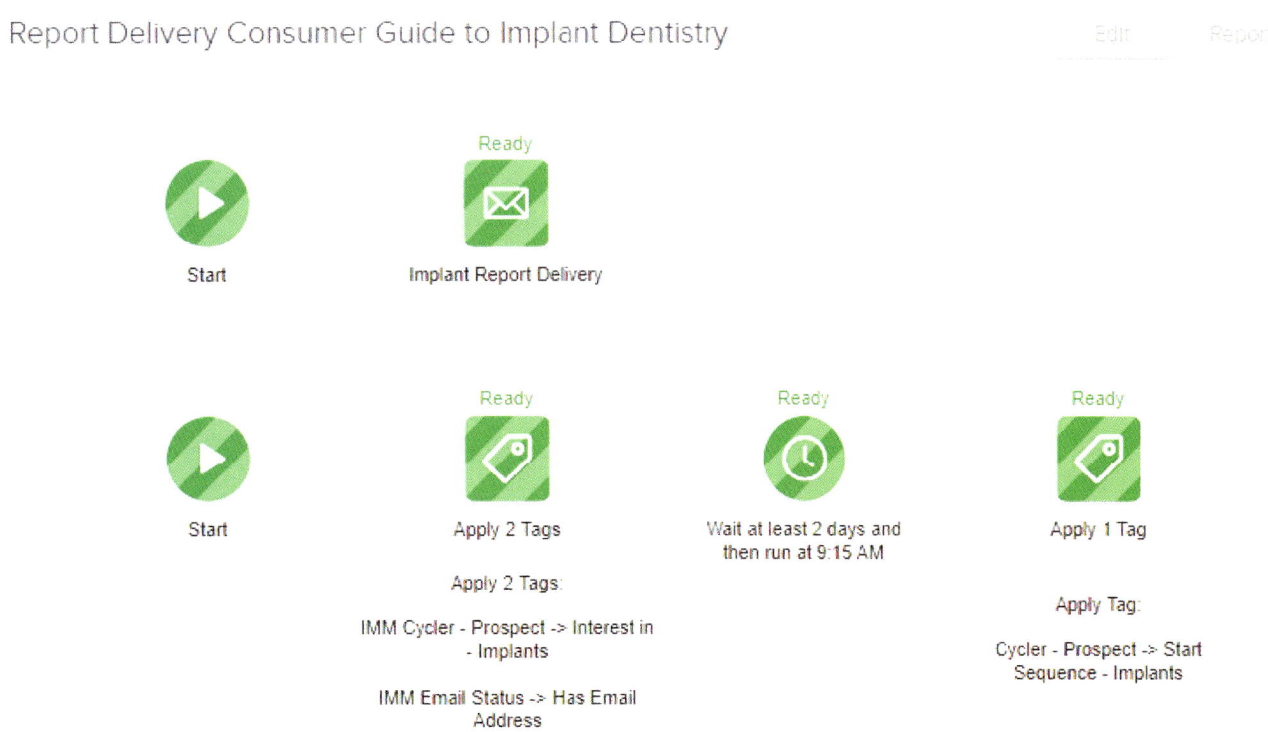

IMPLANT SEMINAR SERIES

The goal of this series is to educate and attract patients. This will help you position yourself as an expert in implant dentistry. This series is an effective way to build your marketing brand and capture referrals.

This includes:

- A print ad. This ad is intended to fit in a newspaper, flyer or circular. The goal is to direct prospects to a landing page where they can sign up for a free report and your seminar.
- A newsletter insert. This is great for your internal e-newsletter or print newsletter or can easily be used in a referring dentist or physician newsletter. The goal is to direct prospects to a landing page where they can sign up for a free report and your seminar.

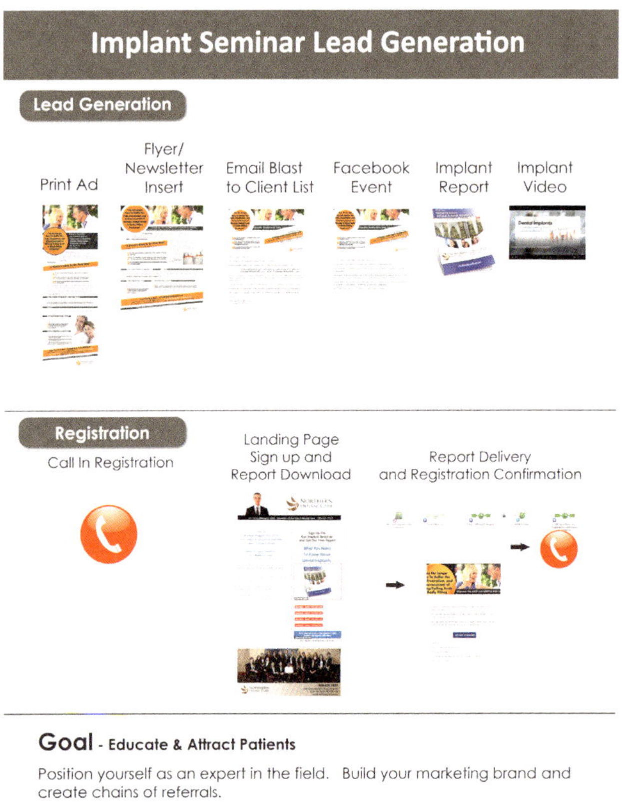

- Email blast invitations. Let everyone on your client and prospect lists know about this informative and valuable event. The goal is to direct them to a landing page where they can sign up for a free report and your seminar.
- Facebook ads. Your prospects are on social media... so you should be too. The goal is to direct them to a landing page where they can sign up for a free report and your seminar.
- A postcard. This gives you away to stand out. In a mailbox full of envelopes, showing up in an alternate format with a well-crafted message and a nice offer makes a difference. The goal is to direct prospects to a landing page where they can sign up for a free report and your seminar.
- Landing page sign up with free report offer. If your prospects end here, it shows your initial push was effective. Your ad, insert or invitation grabbed their attention and led them to the next step—the landing page. Here, you aim to capture their name, email address, phone number, and mailing address and then send them your special report or have them register for your seminar or event.
- Implant report. This is where you speak directly to prospective patients. Explain why they should choose dental implants, why they should choose your office, and why having dental implants placed at your practice is the smartest move they can make to replace their missing teeth.
- Email registration and report delivery follow-up. Once you have contact information, prospects receive a series of emails. The goal of these emails is to acknowledge they've registered for your seminar, let them know the next steps they need to take, educate them, and entice them to contact your office.
- Implant video or PowerPoint presentation. This is a visual version of your report. It is an effective way to connect with those who aren't fans of reading but still want to know more about implant dentistry.

To access swipe files and samples, see the link at the end of the chapter.

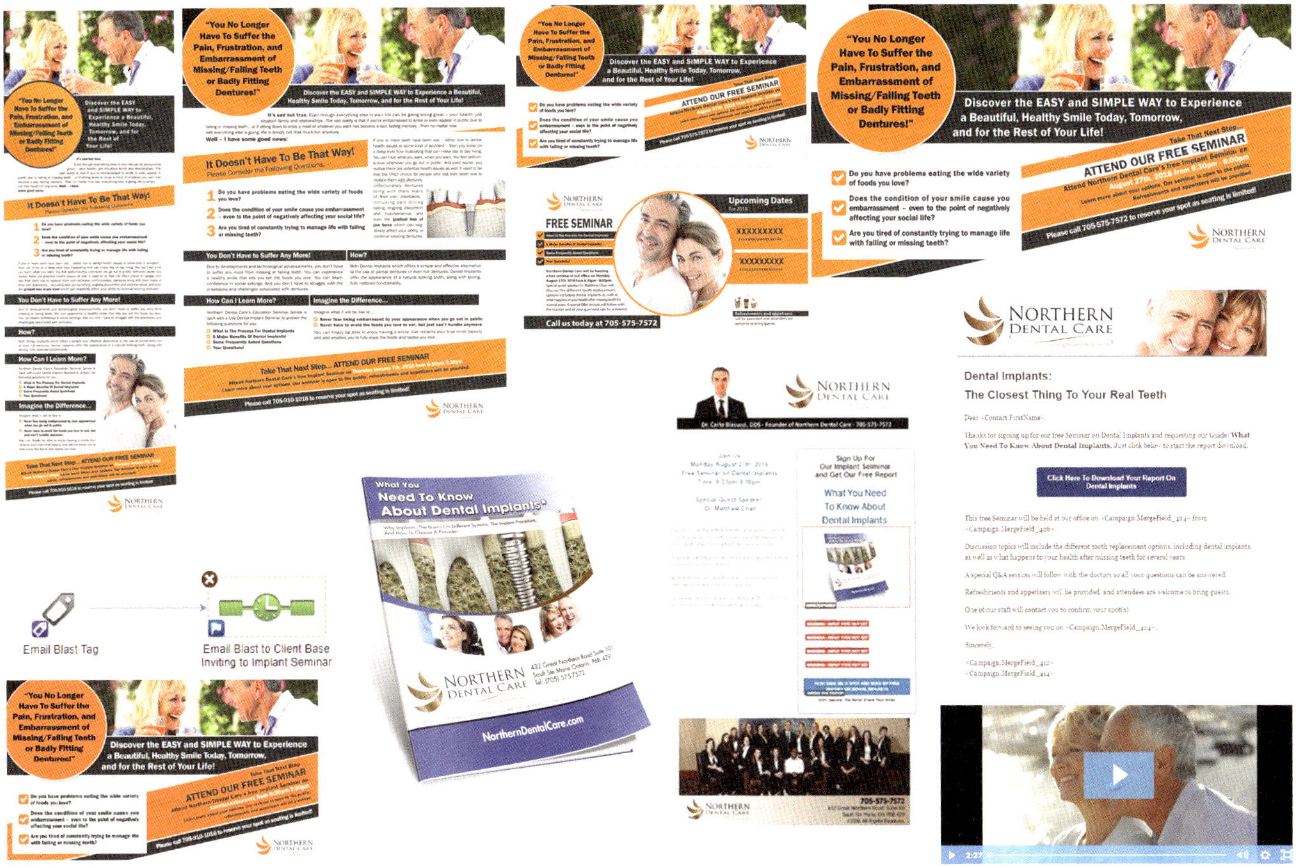
"You No Longer Have To Suffer the Pain, Frustration, and Embarrassment of Missing/Falling Teeth or Badly Fitting Dentures!"
Discover the EASY and SIMPLE WAY to Experience a Beautiful, Healthy Smile Today, Tomorrow, and for the Rest of Your Life!
Northern Dental Care
Dental Implants:
The Closest Thing To Your Real Teeth
Email Blast Tag
Email Blast to Client Base Inviting to Implant Seminar
What You Need To Know About Dental Implants
FREE SEMINAR
Upcoming Dates
Call us today at 705-575-7572

ANXIETY FREE DENTISTRY FUNNEL

The includes:

- A landing page. Gather their information and offer a valuable report that addresses their fears and concerns.
- An anxiety-free dentistry report. Answer their questions and handle their objections in an informative special report that establishes you as the expert in anxiety-free dentistry.
- A report delivery lead prospect email follow-up. Once you have their contact information, prospects receive a series of emails meant to educate them and entice them to contact your office, ready to accept treatment you recommend.

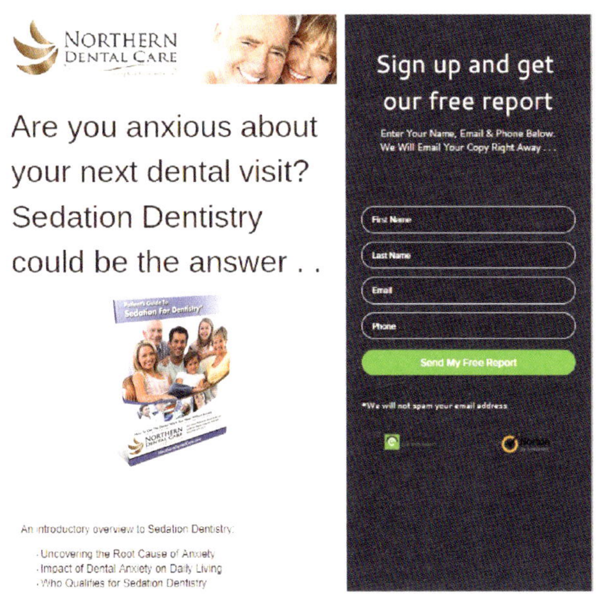

DENTAL PATIENT ENEWSLETTER EMAILS

These weekly or monthly e-newsletters are a way to connect with your patients and prospects. Let them know about special offers at your practice. Tell them about upcoming events. Give them valuable insight about oral hygiene, implants, or whatever you want to share with them. e-newsletters promote top-of-the-mind awareness and let prospects and patients know you care.

To access swipe files and samples, see link at the end of the chapter.

Dental Patient eNewsletter emails

(Created by Dr. Carlo Biasucci, Ontario, Canada)

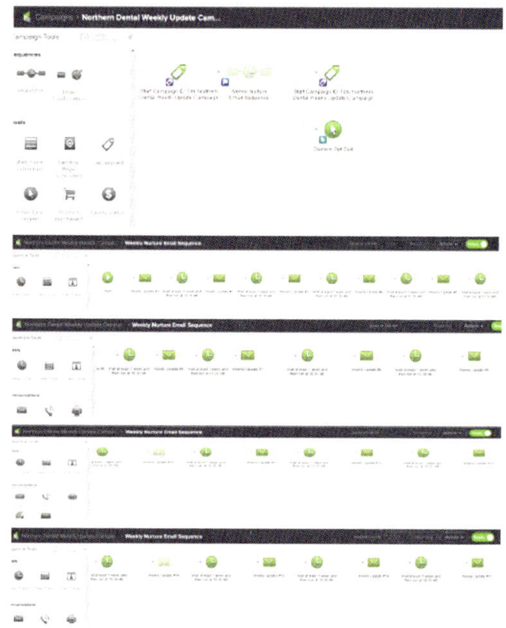

MORE THAN JUST A SMILE BOOK

This is your brag book for your practice—a chance to highlight the exceptional results you achieve for your patients. The first few pages are dedicated to introducing you and the dentists and hygienists who work with you at your practice. Tell your prospective patients a little about what sets you apart. This is the time to brag about your training, awards and accolades. You can mention the advanced tools, technologies and treatment techniques you use in your practice or anything else that sets you apart from all the other dental practices in your area.

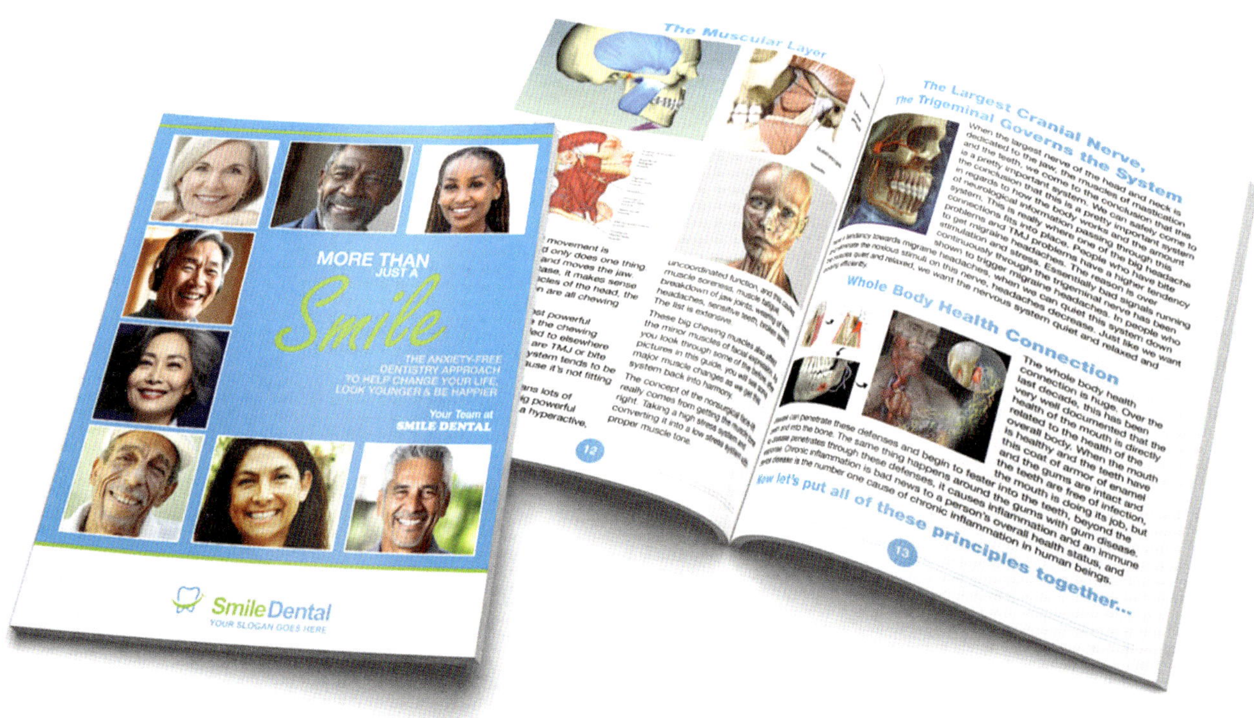

Next, it's time for smiles. Choose a few of your favorite testimonials and case studies. Tell your patients' stories of transformation and include plenty of pictures of smiling faces. Before and after pictures are great here. You want your prospective patients to see the great results you've achieved for patients with teeth in the same shape or worse than their own.

Be sure to discuss how dental implants are more than just cosmetic. This is the time to talk about osseointegration and how dental implants protect the structural integrity of the jawbone. You can talk about how the mouth is an integrated system and the body's first line of defense against harmful bacteria. Stack reason upon reason as to why prospective patients will want to choose dental implants to permanently replace their missing teeth.

COMPLETE DENTAL PHYSICAL CONSULTATION FORMS

Once you have prospective patients in for treatment, your staff needs to know what to do with them. Consultation forms will help any member of your team properly assess prospective patients, gather the information you need, (including medical history), design a treatment plan, and arrange for financing.

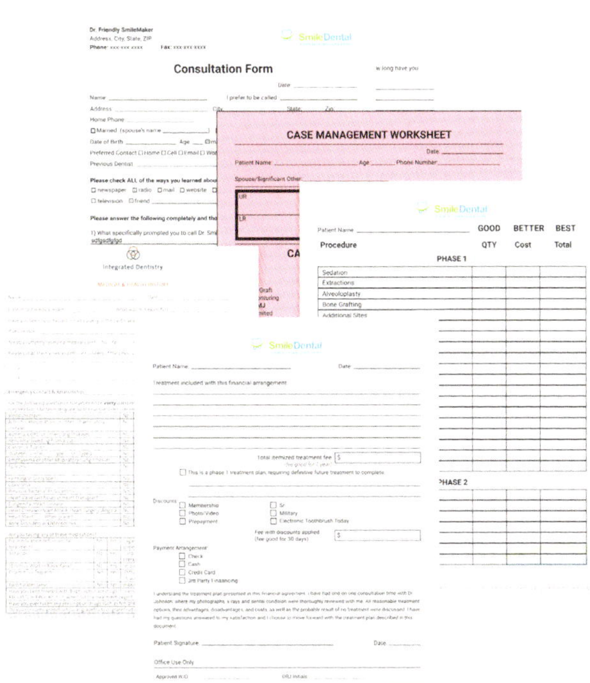

This includes examples of:

- The consultation form
- Case management worksheet
- Combined treatment plan
- Medical history
- Financial arrangement

ORAL-SYSTEM INFOGRAPHICS

These two visuals are a great way to show patients the impact periodontal disease can have on their oral and overall health.

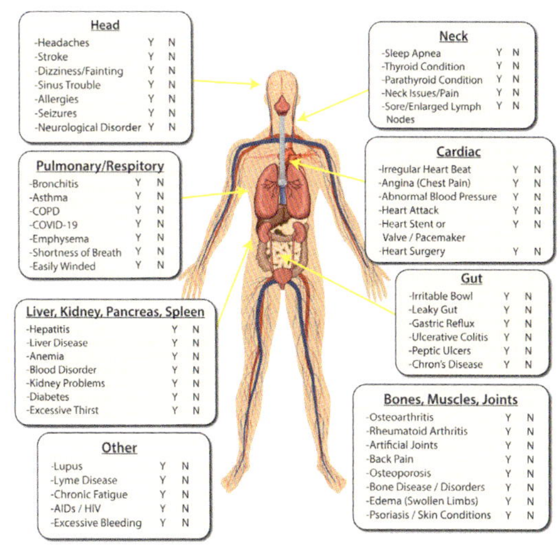

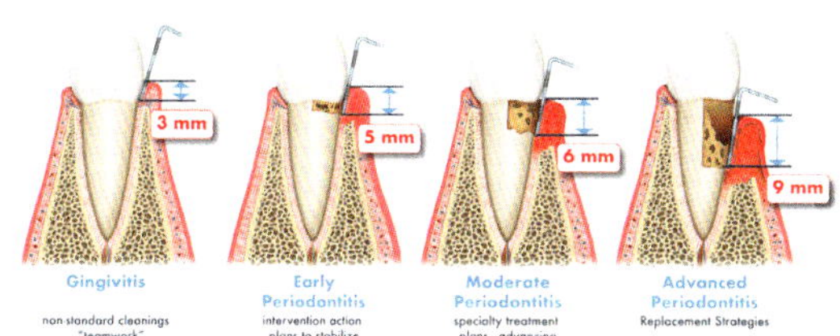

To access swipe files and samples, see the link at end of the chapter.

SHOCK AND AWE

The power of a persuasive shock and awe package cannot be duplicated. This is one of the most effective ways to educate and entice qualified prospects to accept treatment with your practice.

This package includes:

- The folder
- CD label

- Letter
- Shock and awe package with:
  1. A Message from you. This is your chance to speak directly to your prospects. Introduce yourself and your practice. Invite them to become part of your dental family.
  2. An explanation of who depends on your practice. Highlight your ideal patients. Discuss who you care for. More importantly, call out who you want to help the most.
  3. An *Are You Ready?* quiz. Give your prospects the chance to participate. Ask them questions about their oral health and let them answer. When they tally their score, it can be a moment of revelation, where they realize how badly they need dental implants.
  4. An explanation of what happens at your initial consultation. Lay out what they can expect when they come to your office for the first time.
  5. Core products and services. Discuss the treatment you recommend and the in-house services you offer that set you apart from the rest.
  6. Integrated dentistry—continuing smiles. Talk about dentistry as a whole and how your practice can become their dental home, a place to meet their needs and the needs of everyone they love and care about.
  7. Testimonials. Share success stories and let your prospects hear from satisfied patients. Let them see the powerful transformations for themselves.
- Warranty. You stand by your work. Let your prospects know that.

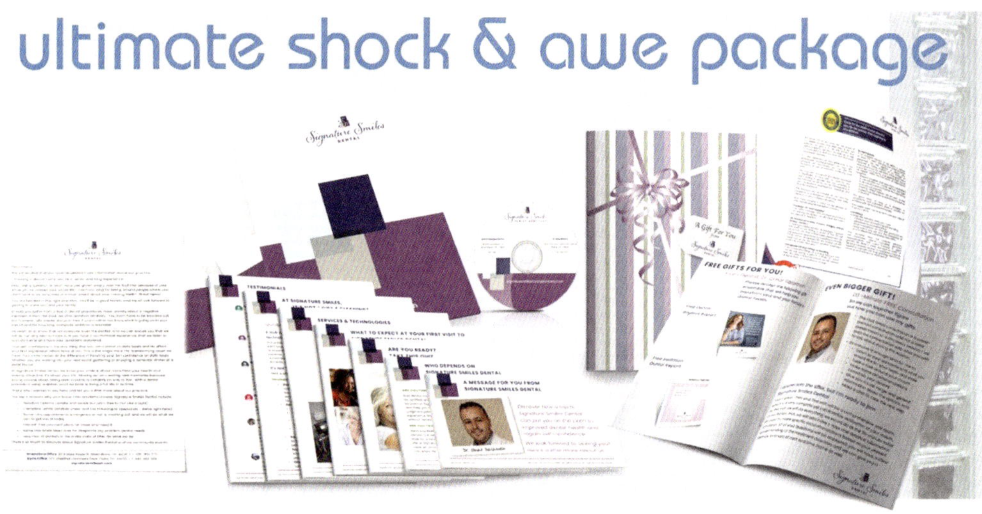

To access swipe files and samples, see the link at end of the chapter.

CASE PRESENTATION

Your case presentation is a way to presell prospects and turn any member of your team into a master salesperson.

This presentation includes:

- A check. Through a discount offer, give them $250 off their treatment when they agree to dental implants.
- A letter to customer. This is a message from you. Here, highlight pain points and offer prospects a permanent solution that you deliver better than anyone else.
- A postcard. This powerful sales message comes in an easy-to-absorb format.
- A step-by-step guide. Walk them through the implant process. Touch on common objections to treatment and blow them out of the water with the benefits they'll receive when they agree to treatment.
- The treatment options. Go over alternate treatments for their missing teeth. Not everyone is a great candidate for implants. Not everyone will be able to afford the treatment you recommend. Here is your chance to discuss alternative tooth replacements while still driving home the point that implants are what you recommend and why.
- Testimonials. Let other satisfied patients tell your story for you. Let them describe the benefits they've experienced thanks to the dental implant treatment they received at your practice.

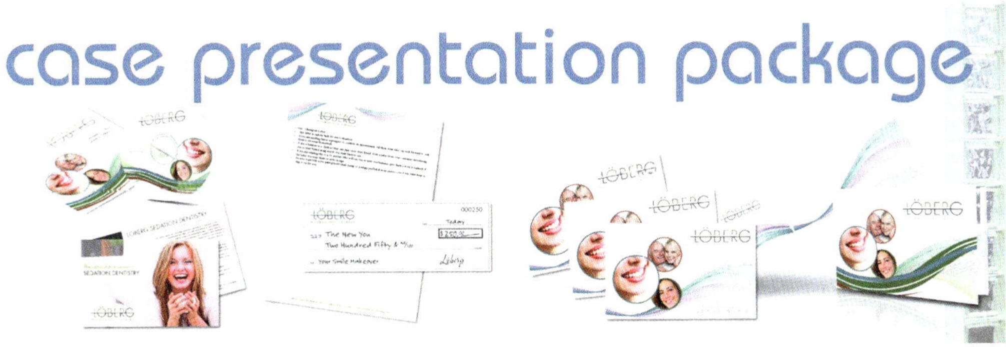

To access swipe files and samples, see the link at end of the chapter.

PRINT ON DEMAND AUTOMATION

A series of follow-up emails and long-term nurture emails, small gifts and letters will keep you on your patients' and prospects' minds. These are great for encouraging repeat business, referrals and top-of-mind awareness.

These include:

- A post appointment follow-up sequence
- Premium long-term nurture (monthly cards and small gifts)
- Classic long-term nurture (monthly greeting cards)
- VIP long-term nurture (2X per year gift and monthly card)

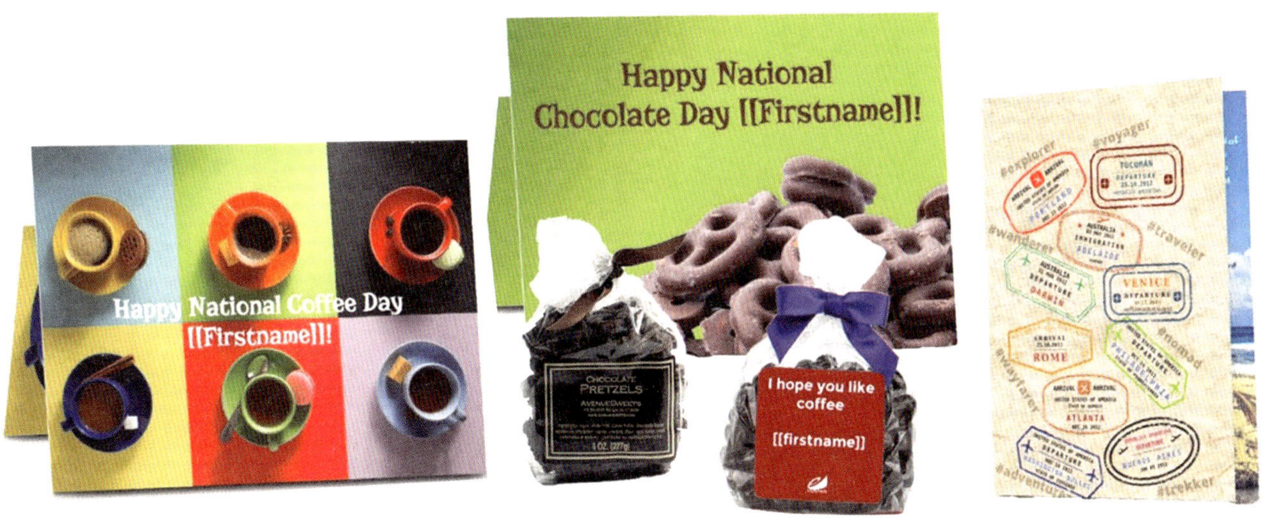
Happy National Coffee Day
[[Firstname]]!
Happy National
Chocolate Day [[Firstname]]!
I hope you like
coffee
[[firstname]]

To access swipe files and samples, see the link at end of the chapter.

IMPLANT AUTOMATED MARKETING

Once prospects make first contact, anything can happen. They can never set an appointment. Set an appointment but fail to show up. Show up but decide not to accept treatment. Or say yes immediately.

These automated marketing sequences cover all bases and include:

- Appointment no set
- Appointment no show
- Appointment no sale
- Neighborhood lead prospect

To access swipe files and samples, see the link at end of the chapter.

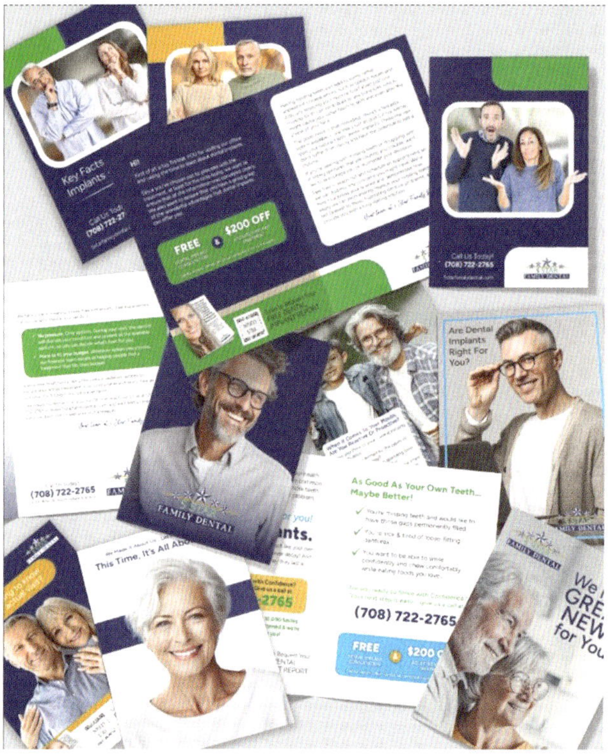

SALES LETTERS

Sales letters delivered to well-qualified prospects in a FedEx envelope are POWERFUL.

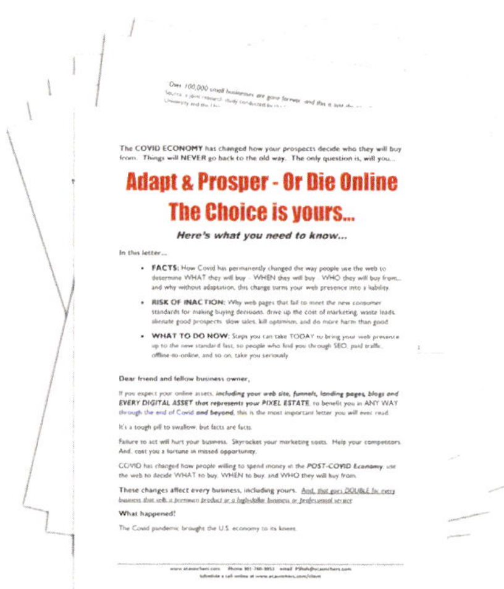

These letters are designed to grab attention and clearly explain why the dental implants you offer at your practice represent the only way prospects will get the results they want with the smile they deserve.

This section includes:

- The main sales letter
- Follow up letter No. 1
- Follow up letter No. 2
- Follow up letter No. 3

My friend, I encourage you to spend time with this chapter. Review each one of these assets. Learn from them and make them your own. And if you would like to learn more about how eLaunchers can put this all to work for your practice, go to www.meetparthiv.com and set an appointment with me. Let's have a conversation. Together, we'll formulate a plan that can launch your practice to a new level of prosperity. Let's see how quickly we can generate your next 100K together.

> *"I always knew there must be at least ONE expert who knew how to do all the advanced list management strategies I wanted done for me...but until I happened upon Parthiv Shaw, I'd not yet MET that person. The AMAZING thing about Parthiv is that he goes way beyond performing what I ask of him. He is at the level where he turns around and asks ME...well, what if...then comes up with BRILLIANT KILLER STRATEGIES that go beyond executing a task at high level. My only hope is that my competition never hears about him!"*
>
> \- Dr. Tom Orent

I look forward to hearing from you.

Sincerely,

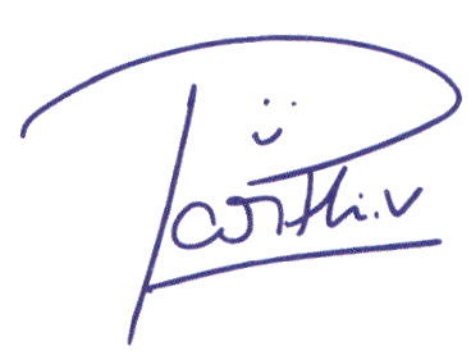

Parthiv Shah

P.S. If you haven't yet visited https://swipefilesandsamples.com be sure to do so to access swipe files and samples from this chapter. Don't want to type? Just scan this QR code:

Acknowledgments

- Dan Kennedy for providing concepts and strategies for business growth. All I have done is take what I learned from him and apply it to dentistry.
- Dipali Shah, CEO of eLaunchers and my lovely wife. Without her love, trust, friendship, and support (emotional, logical, financial) in business and family, I would not be me.
- Dr. Sammy Noumbissi for providing me with the clinical knowledge of implantology and how dental implants work, teaching me the real cost of saying "NO" to recommended care, introducing me to the world of ceramic implantology, and graciously inviting me to the board of the International Academy of Ceramic Implantology (iaoci.com).
- Dr. Chris Phelps for his inspiration and creativity, which gave me the idea to start sellmoreimplants.com, and his ingenuity in dental marketing. Dr. Phelps taught me how to use the power of persuasive words in dentistry and helped me create my implant case presentation package.
- Dr. Derrick Johnson for helping me create the implant patient smile book, a book of stories that became an important part of the implant case presentation package and the take-home implant case treatment plan.
- Dr. John Meis for taking me under his wing and making me a DentalIntel.com power user. Learning how to use DI tools like The Patient Finder gave me the ability to spot pockets of opportunities inside the dental practice database. There are diamonds in your dental database, and Dr. Meis taught me how to mine for them.
- Dr. Carlo Biasucci for implementing EVERYTHING I created for his practice at Northern Dental Care and eventually for all his coaching clients in Canada and the U.S.
- Dr. Dustin Burleson for becoming my first client in the dental coaching industry and bringing me to a portfolio of dentists who hired me.
- Dr. Charles Martin, who taught me how to take what I learned from Dan Kennedy and apply it in dentistry. Dr. Martin also taught me the art and science of "gently soliciting referrals" in dentistry, which worked inside and outside of dentistry for me and my clients. He also taught me how to use Kennedy's shock and awe and sales letters in dentistry.
- Dr. Greg Wych for becoming my FIRST dentist client who painfully experimented with everything I created and applied in his practice.
- Dr. Michael Goldberg for introducing me to the concept of the oral-systemic connection and teaching me how to build a bond between dentists and physicians to provide comprehensive care for patients inside and outside their mouth. Dr. Goldberg taught me how to work with medical billing companies to help seek reimbursement for significant dentistry from patients' medical insurance.
- Master copywriter Russell Martino for being my scribe, my friend, my philosopher, my guide and my inspiration. Without his guidance and advice, I would not be a prolific author with more than a dozen books and a patent.
- Clate Mask, CEO of Keap.com, for his direct, personal involvement in my professional journey in marketing automation. Without it, what I have accomplished would not have been possible. My entire marketing automation engine, including the Business Kamasutra campaign and the internal marketing machine for dentists, is built exclusively on the Keap.com application.

- Justin Biggs, CEO of mailboxpower.com, who built a print automation engine that automates the entire dental patient experience in print, making it possible for every dentist to send something in print at every milestone for every patient, before, during and after treatment.
- The marketing, sales and product development teams behind Dental Intelligence software (dentalintel.com). This is the engine that helps dentists look at the data and see what is working and what is not working in their practice. This is my software of choice for my "dental economics" work.
- Terrie Angela Lopez for taking my thoughts in raw format and articulating them in a way the world can understand. Terrie has the ability to take the spirit of my brand and display it in a human-friendly way. Without her being my scribe, I would be a non-charismatic genius who would be dismissed without being understood.

About the Author

Sell-More-Implants™ (and Dental Growth Machine) are Powered By eLaunchers, a business growth agency. We specialize in developing powerful brands.

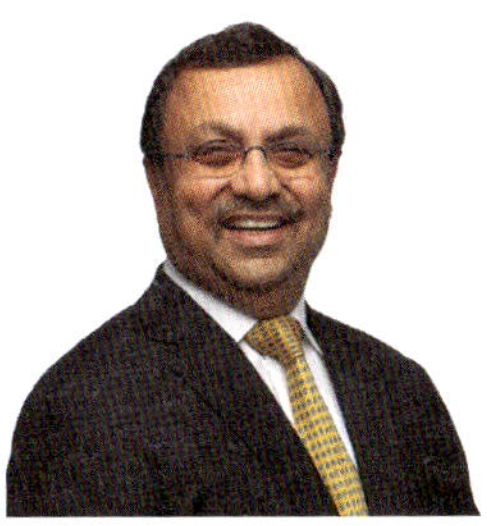

The very hands-on CEO and Founder of eLaunchers and developer of Sell-More-Implants™ is Parthiv Shah. After serving in the Indian Air Force, Parthiv immigrated to America, earned an MBA in Marketing, and has worked in direct-response marketing for over 30 years. He is a True American Success Story, having started a unique marketing services company from scratch and build it to pre-eminence in the field. You can read the complete "My Story – by Parthiv Shah" at the end of this insert, but here is what you most need to know in brief:

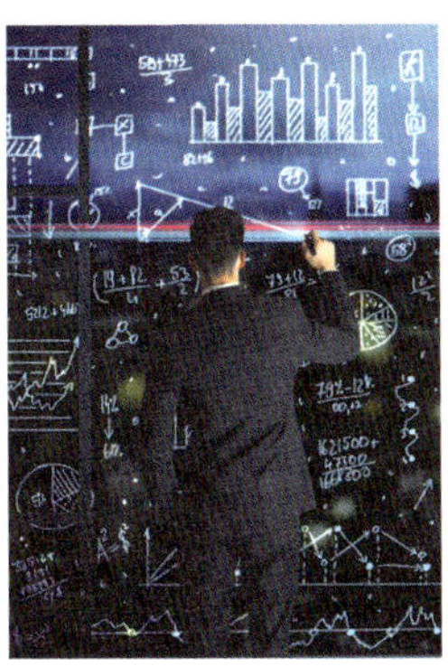

Parthiv is, first and foremost, a data scientist. He "looks into" your practice and patient information and "sees" what you can't, with the naked eye. Using highly sophisticated data-mining, modeling, and matching tools, he is, quite simply, able to find and extract "stored value" inside your past and present, inactive and active patient records, as well as past and current leads that you cannot do on your own, with "the naked eye."

Second, Parthiv Shah is a direct-response marketing specialist. He has studied all the works and strategies of over 100 leaders in this field, including Dan Kennedy, Jay Abraham, Seth Godin, Russell Brunson, and Brian Kurtz, and he has invested well over $1million in his focused education. Parthiv is also the author of 12 books. Since 2001, he has applied all this knowledge directly to dental practices. The Sell-More-Implants™ System is his latest breakthrough.

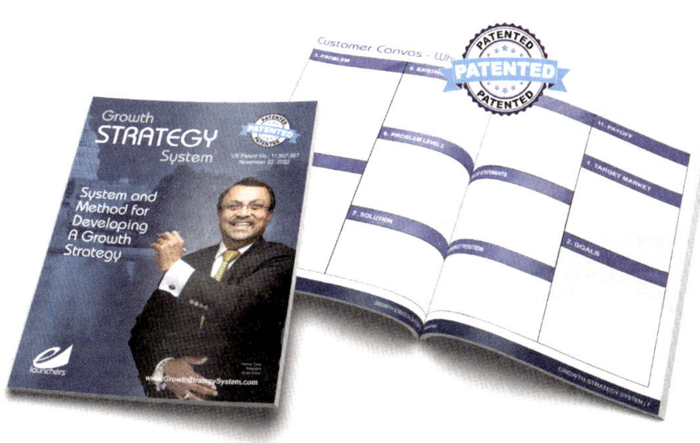

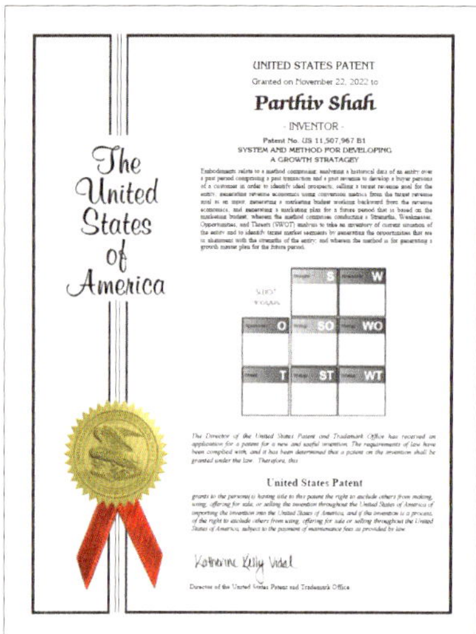

His scientific marketing is so unusual and exceptionally effective that he has been granted U.S. PATENT #11,507,967 for his unique method of SWOT ANALYSIS (Strengths, Weaknesses, Opportunities, Threats) and for developing Growth Strategies.

Third, Parthiv owns eLaunchers, a certified implementation agency for HubSpot, Keap, and Mailbox Power, specializing in customer relations and marketing automation. Parthiv uses sophisticated tools and technologies like Dental Intel, Databox, IDI, and others. In 2022, Parthiv won his second 2CC award from ClickFunnels and has built over 450 funnels on ClickFunnels.

Parthiv has mailed over a BILLION pieces of direct mail, worked for over 1,000 clients (dentists and non-dentists), and worked on more than 10,000 direct marketing projects.

Fourth, Parthiv is famously a very hard worker!

Read his MY STORY and you'll see why! Ryan Deiss, Founder of DIGITAL MARKETER says: "Parthiv is the hardest working man in America!"

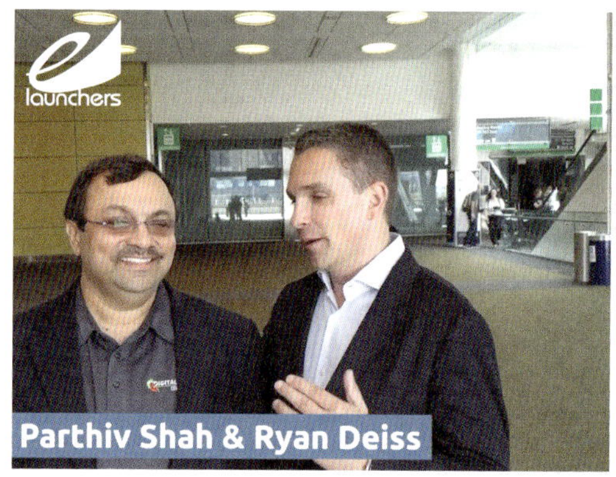

Parthiv Shah & Ryan Deiss

Fifth and final point, Parthiv has a stellar reputation within both the dental and among dental industry leaders. Parthiv's exceptional expertise and unique contributions to practice growth have been recognized by dental industry leaders, including Dr. Tom Orent, Dr. John Meiss, Dr. Dustin Burleson, Dr. Christopher Phelps, Dr. Carlo Biasucci, and others. He also serves as a Board Member of the International Academy of Ceramic Implantology (IAOC).

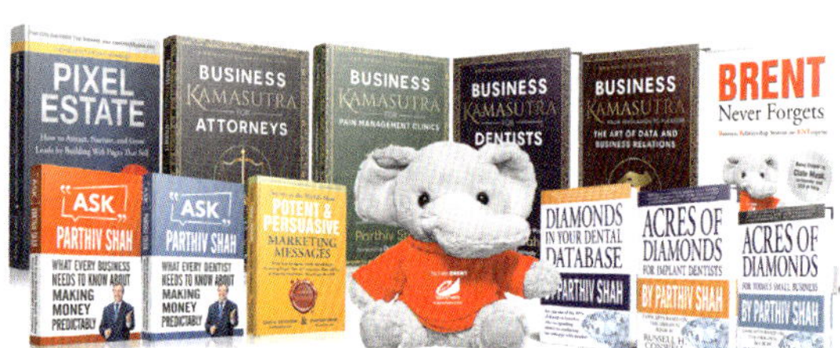

Parthiv is the author of over a dozen books including BUSINESS KAMASUTRA FOR DENTISTS, BRENT Never Forgets, Pixel Estate, and others.

His team at eLaunchers.com includes data analysts, direct- response copywriters, digital marketing content creators, graphic designers, marketing technology implementation experts, web developers, funnel builders, and other specialists. ALL client work is done under Parthiv's direct, personal supervision. YOU will receive Parthiv's personal attention and work with him personally– you will NOT be shunted off to wet-behind-the-ears techies in Dilbert™ cubicles who know nothing about dental practice.

MY STORY – BY PARTHIV SHAH

The level of sophistication and science behind the Sell-More-Implants™ System has typically been affordable only by large corporations and has been their business advantage. By developing a System whose costs are effectively shared by hundreds of individual practices (limited to one per area), we are able to provide the same competitive advantage to independently owned private practices. In an era of expanding and intensifying corporate competition, this is especially important.

OUR METHODS ARE SO UNIQUE AND INNOVATIVE THAT WE HAVE BEEN AWARDED A U.S. PATENT FOR OUR SYSTEMS!

Only ***six*** *patents have*
ever *been granted for "Business Growth Strategies," and ours is the first since 2013.*

To obtain this patent, we had to ***prove*** *three things:*
that we had something ***unique,*** *something* ***useful,***
and a functioning ***"system"*** *(noy just an "idea").*

WE WILL PUT OUR PATENTED SYSTEM TO WORK FOR YOU!

I came to America in 1989 and settled my multi-generational family in the suburbs of Boston. While in the Indian Air Force, I became fascinated with computers. One of my core job duties was to type in the "daily orders" and then stencil print them out on a good old-fashioned dot-matrix printer (without ribbons), which I would then duplicate on something called a Cyclostyle Duplicator. This was my first exposure to "mass communications"!

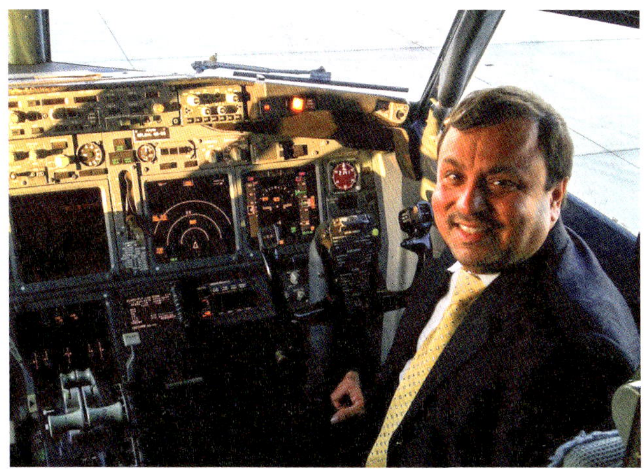

My first job in the United States was in marketing for a health club. After generating multiple leads in high foot-traffic locations, I would cold-call interested potential members. I discovered that I was pretty good at it—and I actually liked it! Consequently, I was successful at generating many sales.

jmperrone

I soon moved on to work for a direct mail marketing firm, J.M. Perrone Company in Hingham, MA, where I introduced a software product called Telemagic to senior management. They adopted it for their operations. While my coworkers laughed and told me that learning the system was a huge waste of time, I soon convinced them that the software, along with the computer, was like owning a "Thousand Dollar Rolodex". The owner of the company, a Professor at Bentley College in Boston, encouraged me to go after my MBA in Marketing, which I completed at Bentley College in 1994. During my studies, I wrote many papers on Direct Marketing, Database Marketing, and Direct Mail Marketing. One of the assignments in a New Product Development class was to create a product and a marketing plan. I developed a mailing list to the Indian community in America. This was my first introduction to data-based marketing.

Over the next 12 years, I continued to develop and expand my skills in Customer Relationship Management (CRM) implementation, with my company investing heavily in my ongoing education.

As I took on greater responsibilities, I decided to make it easier to find potential clients by becoming my own resident list expert. I soon realized that I could provide a needed service to our clients, so I began a program to buy and sell data on their behalf.

In 1998, I started a dot-com company, but the business failed miserably. Broke and deep in debt, I returned to my old company and asked for my job back, and even convinced my boss to give me a substantial raise to help pay off my debts. He gave me a short leash, but I was well rewarded when, almost immediately, I closed a $400,000 deal with Children's Hospital. I was back on track, but like most entrepreneurs, I got the bug to strike out on my own again.

In 2002, I opened Listlaunchers, Boston's premier list brokerage company, assisting the printing industry, direct mail companies, and telemarketing firms. From this I learned a dynamic new way of printing content: digitizing offset printing jobs, which significantly boosted profitability. Jobs that previously sold for $7,500 were now selling for over $12,000. Our sales tripled in three years.

In 2005, I sold Listlaunchers for multi-seven figures and became part of a larger conglomerate. Unfortunately, a failed business transaction that left me and my family in debt once again.

My business, Listlaunchers, was killed... but I survived!

list launchers

In 2006, starting over once again, I founded eLaunchers.com. The difference this time was that I knew exactly what I was doing. I took everything I had learned about marketing, technology, list generation, success, and failure and rolled it into one super dynamic company.

The years from 2006 to 2009 were trying times, a struggle to make ends meet. In 2009, I accidentally stumbled upon a local GKIC study club. I joined their program, bought various books and courses taught by Bill Glazer and Dan Kennedy. Over time, I became an expert at implementing Dan Kennedy's concepts.

In 2011, while attending a Dan Kennedy's event in Cleveland, I was approached during a break by a good-looking guy who said: "Hi Parthiv, I have been following you for a while and watching you work with others. I like you; I am ready to get started with you." That person was **Dr. Dustin Burleson**. I began working for Dr. Burleson's practice, and during a visit to Maryland for a one-day consultation, he asked me if I would be kind enough to go to Richmond with him to attend **Dr. Charles Martin's** mastermind. It was there that I met my friend **Dr. Greg Wych**. Dr. Martin was the first in the group to hire me, followed by Dr. Wych and then several others.

Eventually Dr. Burleson started a coaching program for orthodontists, and I became the implementation expert for his members.

Prior to that, I worked with **Dr. Tom Orent** as his list research and market segmentation strategist, where I developed a multi-step, short-run direct mail program for dentists and a dental patient newsletter initiative.

This is my story. It is a classic entrepreneur's journey: starting with little or nothing, turning it into something, then back again to nothing and then rebuilding it into something successful. The difference this time is that *I have not only bounced back, but I do not have to–and will not–waiver from my successful formula! I will show you what I know so you can achieve greater success than ever before.*

That is a snapshot of my business background and the experiences that led me to conceive my "dream." Today, I own a multinational technology firm with offices in three countries and a team of technologists, programmers, system architects, designers, writers, marketers, and operations professionals—each driven by a shared passion for one thing: RESULTS!

Book Your Call Today

at www.meetparthiv.com

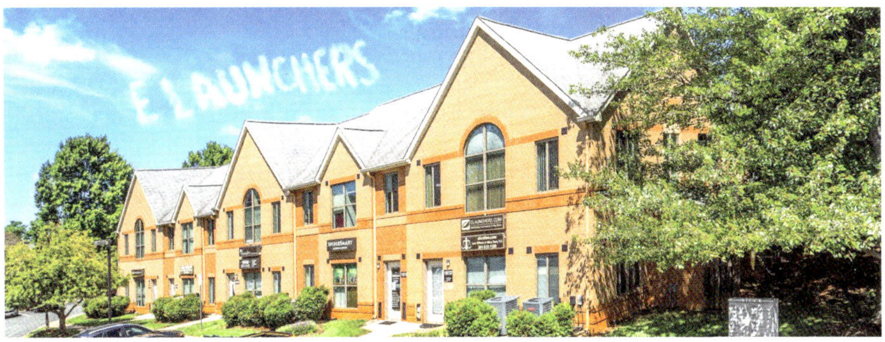

SellMoreImplants.com

Powered by eLaunchers

Since 2002, Hundreds of Clients,
Thousands of Campaigns, and Billions of Pieces Mailed

Parthiv Shah, eLaunchers.com
13236 Executive Park Terrace
Germantown, MD 20874
301.760.3953
pshah@elaunchers.com